Step by Step Management of Equinus Foot by Ilizarov Technique

Step by Step
Management of Equinus Foot by Ilizarov Technique

R.A. Agrawal
MS (Ortho)
Director
Agrawal Orthopaedic Hospital
Gorakhpur, Uttar Pradesh

Emeritus Prof. Sureshwar Pandey
MBBS (Hons), MS, FICS, MS (Ortho), FIAMS, FAC, FAS, FACS, FNAMS
Ex-Head of the Department
Department of Orthopaedics
Rajendra Medical College, Ranchi, Jharkand

Prof. Ustiantsev Vasilli Ivanovich
MD
Clinical Director
The Federal Scientific Practical Centre of
Medico-Social Expertise and Rehabilitation of the Invalids
Moscow (Russia)

Contact Address:
Agrawal Orthopaedic Hospital
Jubilee Road, Gorakhpur, UP, India
Tel. 91-551-2333102, 2349789
Email: agrawalram@hotmail.com   Website: www.aohospital.org

JAYPEE BROTHERS
MEDICAL PUBLISHERS (P) LTD.
New Delhi

Published by

Jitendar P Vij
Jaypee Brothers Medical Publishers (P) Ltd
EMCA House, 23/23B Ansari Road, Daryaganj
New Delhi 110 002, India
Phones: +91-11-23272143, +91-11-23272703, +91-11-23282021, +91-11-23245672
Fax: +91-11-23276490, +91-11-23245683   e-mail: jaypee@jaypeebrothers.com
Visit our website: www.jaypeebrothers.com

Branches

- 2/B Akruti Society, Jodhpur Gam Road, Satellite
  Ahmedabad 380 015, Phone: +91-079-30988717

- 202 Batavia Chambers, 8 Kumara Krupa Road, Kumara Park East,
  Bangalore 560 001, Phones: +91-80-22285971, +91-80-22382956, +91-80-30614073
  Tele Fax: +91-80-22281761   e-mail: jaypeemedpubbgl@eth.net

- 282 IIIrd Floor, Khaleel Shirazi Estate, Fountain Plaza
  Pantheon Road, **Chennai** 600 008, Phones: +91-44-28262665, +91-44-28269897
  Fax: +91-44-28262331   e-mail: jpchen@eth.net

- 4-2-1067/1-3, Ist Floor, Balaji Building, Ramkote
  Cross Road, **Hyderabad** 500 095, Phones: +91-40-55610020, +91-40-24758498
  Fax: +91-40-24758499   e-mail: jpmedpub@rediffmail.com

- 1A Indian Mirror Street, Wellington Square, **Kolkata** 700 013,
  Phones: +91-33-22456075, +91-33-22451926 Fax: +91-33-22456075
  e-mail: jpbcal@cal.vsnl.net.in

- 106 Amit Industrial Estate, 61 Dr SS Rao Road, Near MGM Hospital
  Parel, **Mumbai** 400 012, Phones: +91-22-24124863, +91-22-24104532, +91-22-30926896
  Fax: +91-22-24160828   e-mail: jpmedpub@bom7.vsnl.net.in
  e-mail: jpmedpub@bom7.vsnl.net.in

- "KAMALPUSHPA", 38 Reshimbag, Opp. Mohota Science College, Umred Road
  Nagpur 440 009, Phones: +91-712-3945220, +91-712-2704275
  e-mail: jpnagpur@rediffmail.com

Step by Step Management of Equinus Foot by Ilizarov Technique

First Edition: **2006**

ISBN 81-8061-710-6

Typeset at   JPBMP typesetting unit
Printed at   Paras Offset Pvt. Ltd., C-176, N.I.A., Phase-1, New Delhi

Preface

A deformity in whatever form, at whichever site, and in whatever age is not acceptable by any one. Not surprisingly, in the pre-civilization era, the disabled persons were put to crucible tests for survivorship, i.e. if they could work hard, earn their livelihood and help their community in their needs, then only they had the right to survive. On the other hand, those who could not prove their worth on the above fronts were done to death. Deformities produce physical disfigurement and physical disabilities. It also produces psychological depression, needs more energy consumption in executing even the routine functions and subsequently it leads to secondary deformities locally and even distantly resulting into ultimate premature degenerative changes in various joints. Therefore, any deformity must be corrected as far as possible.

With the dawn of the civilization, the disabled persons started to expect their right to survive in the world. Gradually, society started to accept them, treat them, rehabilitate them and provide them the dignity of life. Ultimately, the medical world took the challenge of preventing, managing and rehabilitating these disabled/deformed persons. There has been variable success on all fronts. However, the maximum success has been achieved in correcting the deformity and minimizing the deformity. In this very direction, the birth of the "third dimension (rehabilitation medicine) of medicine" took place. Most of the initial deformities are amenable to controlled, graduated, stretching schedule and proper physiotherapy. However, as the deformities advance, they become stiff and some semi-invasive or invasive method for management has to be employed.

The old standard treatment methods include plaster wedge technique; percutaneous, subtotal / total tenotomy; and taking care of other deforming tissues. Beyond that, surgeries on tendon and / or bones and joints help a lot in correcting the deformity. The introduction of 3-D pictures of any deformed and corresponding normal portion helps a lot in deciding the modality and time factor in bringing the normal architecture in that region of the limb.

In this very direction, the Kurgan surgeon G.A. Ilizarov introduced his technique for tackling various problems and one of them has been for the correction of fixed deformity. The principle behind Ilizarov technique has great depth. However, against the speed with which Ilizarov technique was accepted all over the world, its decline unfortunately is also being palpably observed. There can be several reasons but its overuse, uncalculated use, misuse and under-use have a definite role to play for its decline. And nonetheless the improper passing of K-wire, injudicious selection of point of entry of wires and improper placement of rings have a definite role to play in bringing disrepute to Ilizarov technique. Let us not blame the young enthusiastic surgeons who want to master any technology in minimum time and minimum effort. We feel there is hardly any monograph detailing the basics of Ilizarov technique, which includes acquaintance with the hardware, proper selection of patient, pin-pointing the placement of the K-wires and the direction of the wire advancement.

The biomechanics itself is a tough subject and we want to avoid intricacies of the biomechanics in our practical life. However, the understanding of the basic kinematics, anatomical localization of the suitable points and basic physiology of execution of function are mandatory before attempting to master any technique.

We have tried to tackle the above problems in a lucid and descriptive manner so that this manual may be useful even to the beginners who want to know, learn, execute and get effective result after the use of the Ilizarov technique.

We all want to put our best to make this monograph acceptable by all, however, there may be many shortcomings for which apology is solicited.

In preparing this monograph we have consulted many books and journals, derived in ideas and inspiration and have been educated through different sources. However, we are particularly indebted to the books given in bibliography which we have consulted several times. We have no hesitation in giving full credit to these sources. We acknowledge the constant help of our sincere colleagues and friends like Dr. S.S. Jha, Dr. Anil Juyal, Dr. Anuj Jain, Dr. B.L. Agrawal, Dr. Mukesh Chandra, Dr. R.C. Srivastava, Dr. K.N. Mishra PT, Dr. Pradeep, Mr. Arun, Mr. Girja Shankar, Mr. Anoop, Er. D.N. Srivastava, Mr. Sajjad, Mr. Ajay and Mr. Shankar Joshi. The typing, aligning the manuscript and improving the script is the real tough job in preparing any book—and all that have been done tirelessly by Mr. Shyam Ji Srivastava who remained alert and active for this work at all the time.

The authors could not have concentrated on the work unless the family members had provided them full cooperation. And to this, the dear family of Dr. R.A. Agrawal has stood the test of time accepting all the eccentricities during the preparation of this book. The contribution of Dr. R.A. Agrawal's wife Mrs. Rashmi, son Dr. Rajat, the young budding of orthopaedic surgeon and daughter Miss. Richa, the software engineer simply deserve all credit in uninterrupted production of this book.

Dr. R.A. Agrawal
Prof. Sureshwar Pandey
Prof. Ustiantsev Vasilli Ivanovich

Prolog

The deformities, anywhere in the body right from head to foot, throw an exciting challenge for correction. However, the foot and ankle deformities pose further problems because of their strategic location at the base of the body for receiving, distributing and propelling the weight both in stance and locomotion.

There can be several causes of deformities but the more common are congenital, paralytic, traumatic, infective and neurogenic disorders. Of these, congenital and paralytic ones are most common.

Paralytic foot deformities are either due to flaccid paralysis such as in poliomyelitis, traumatic paraplegia or spastic problems as seen in cerebral palsy, residual hemiplegia, etc. The foot deformities are hardly in one plane, since multiplaner and multiaxial involvements automatically creep-in the process of development and progression of deformity. Proper understanding of the planes and biomechanics of normal foot and ankle, and proper analysis of pathodynamics of deformity(ies) are quite essential before contemplating to correct any type of deformity.

There have been many methods and techniques to correct the deformity of the foot but none is fullproof and several limitations and complications have been encountered in the process of correction, to mention a few — problems in skin closure, neurovascular problems, infections, stiffness, leg length discrepancy, etc. All are notorious to tackle but the management of neurovascular problems and leg length discrepancy are more demanding.

Conventional management of the deformity usually consists of gradual stretching, plaster wedge correction and operative interference and like tendon transfer procedures, tenotomy, osteotomy, stabilization and fusion of the joints. However, the advent of Ilizarov technology ushered in a new hope of dynamic correction of these deformities, albeit with the associated shortcomings like prolonged treatment, bulky hardware, pin tract infection and difficult proper patient compliance.

If done, after properly analyzing the pathodynamics of the deformity compared to the normal biomechanics, the Ilizarov technology has a definite edge over other methods as enumerated above. The basic principle of Ilizarov methodology is gradual and controlled stretching of the soft tissues which induces minimal fibrosis and thus, recurrence of the deformity is minimized with proper preoperative planning, preconstruction of the frames, insertion of wires, selection of rings, fixation of rods, postoperative monitoring and inducing steps to gain the patient's compliance, ultimate results are more gratifying.

Though, Ilizarov technique became acceptable all over the globe in comparatively short period, its acceptability is gradually dwindling. There may be several factors but one factor appears apparent that probably there is no monograph detailing the exact basic procedure for selecting the proper patient and handling the instrument and selecting and positioning the wires according to the various indications. The present monograph is an initial attempt to outline the basic procedure of Ilizarov technique in different corrective procedures of different deformities. This monograph has been prepared with a mind to simplify the practical procedure involved in managing the equinus deformity of the foot by Ilizarov method.

Contents

CD Content

Correction of Equinus Deformity by Ilizarov

Chapter 1

Planes and Biomechanics of Foot

GROSS UNDERSTANDING OF PLANES AND BIOMECHANICS OF FOOT

In any three-dimensional assessment, three planes have to be considered and this holds true for the ankle and foot as well. The three planes are:

1. Sagittal
2. Horizontal
3. Frontal or coronal.

While describing any deformity, usually the first two planes are considered. Besides these planes, rotational deformities are assessed against certain axis, which exist separately for each movement.

In a human being with bipedal locomotion, the biomechanics of the foot has been oriented to serve the basic and refined functions of the foot. The basic functions of the foot are:

1. To receive the weight of the body
2. To distribute the weight throughout the foot
3. To help in locomotion in bipedal fashion
4. To provide soundless springing gait
5. To execute fine functions like dancing, gymnastic activities etc.

To achieve all the above goals, minimal requirement is the plantigrade foot, in which the weight is borne by different parts of the foot in a systematic order. There have been several opinions about the weight distribution in the foot but the most accepted opinion is in the following way. Unit-wise, if the body weight is 24 units then each foot receives 12 units, of these 12 units 50 percent, i.e. 6 units are borne by the hindfoot and 6 by the forefoot in which 2 units are borne by the ball of great toe and 1 each for other toes. The midfoot is mainly concerned about dynamic distribution of the weight mainly through the medial longitudinal arch. From hindfoot, the weight is transmitted to the forefoot in a piano-distribution pattern mainly through the transverse arches.

Any deviation from this plantigrade pattern will lead to deformity(ies) in the foot.

BROAD UNDERSTANDING OF DIFFERENT DEFORMITIES OF ANKLE–FOOT IN TERMS OF PLANES (Figure 1.1)

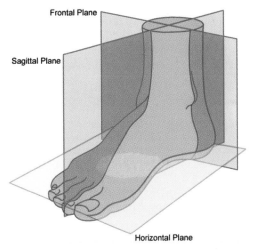

FIGURE 1.1: 3-D picture of foot showing planes

Table 1.1: Planes and deformities

Planes and different deformities	Seat of deformity	Remarks
1. Sagittal plane		

a. Equinus
b. Equinocavus—
   Clawing of toes
c. Pes planus—
   Flat foot
d. Calcaneus
	Ankle hindfoot, midfoot, forefoot	

2. Frontal plane		
a. Varus of heel b. Valgus of heel	Deformity of hindfoot	To be viewed from back
3. Horizontal plane		
a. Adduction of forefoot b. Abduction of forefoot	Deformity of forefoot	To be viewed from up-down
4. Supination		
a. Plantar flexion at ankle b. Varus of heel c. Cavus of midfoot d. Adduction of forefoot	Ankle, hindfoot midfoot, forefoot	
5. Pronation		
a. Dorsiflexion at ankle b. Valgus of heel c. Collapse arch at midfoot d. Abduction of forefoot	Ankle, hindfoot midfoot, forefoot	

Sagittal Plane Deformities

This plane is visualized when we see the deformity from the side. The main deformities in this plane are shown in Figures 1.2 to 1.5.

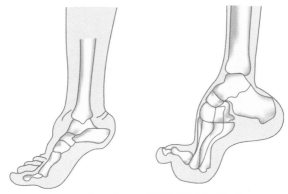

FIGURE 1.2: Equinus foot   **FIGURE 1.3:** Equinocavus foot

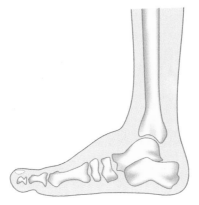

FIGURE 1.4: Pes Planus (Flat) foot

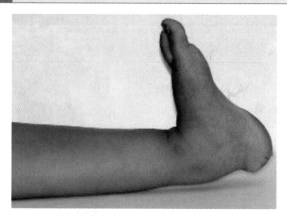

FIGURE 1.5: Calcaneus foot

Frontal Plane Deformities

The main deformities in this plane are shown in Figures 1.6 and 1.7.

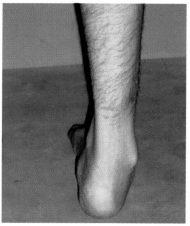

FIGURE 1.6: Varus heel

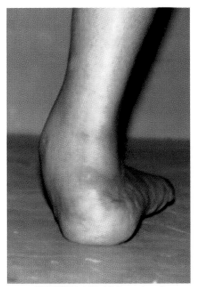

FIGURE 1.7: Valgus heel
(Note Valgus elements at ankle
and subtalar joint)

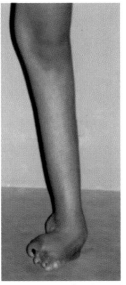

FIGURE 1.8: Supinated
foot

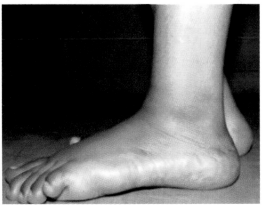

FIGURE 1.9: Pronated foot

Horizontal Plane Deformities

The main deformities in this plane are shown in Figures 1.10 to 1.12.

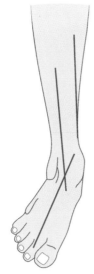

FIGURE 1.10: Abducted foot

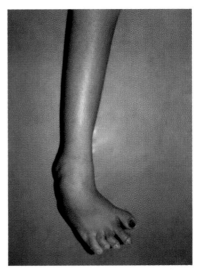

FIGURE 1.11: Adducted foot (dorsal view)

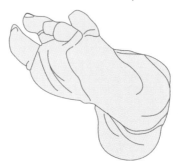

FIGURE 1.12: Adducted foot (Plantar view)

Chapter 2

Equinus Deformity

UNDERSTANDING ABOUT THE EQUINUS DEFORMITY

Historically, the recorded or depicted evidence of 'Equinus' deformity is difficult to trace, but for the evidence of equino–varus deformity of right foot of the mummy of Pharoan of Siptah of the nineteenth dynasty has been kept in the Egyptian museum (Pandey 1990) (Figures 2.1 and 2.2).

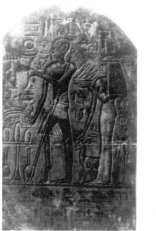 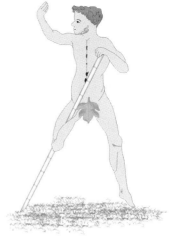

FIGURES 2.1 and 2.2: Equino-varus deformity of right foot has been evidenced from the mummy of Pharoan of Siptah. The figures are preserved in the Egyptian museum

Since the core concern of this monograph is equinus deformity, we will like to concentrate on pathodynamics of the equinus deformity. The term 'equinus' deformity has derived its name from the foot pattern of the horse (Latin—'*equinus*' means horse), in which weight is borne only by the forefoot.

To avoid the dilemma about the description of the equinus deformity, it appears worthwhile to understand the following descriptive terms. The normal range of pure dorsiflexion at ankle is 20° and the plantar flexion is 45°.

1. From zero position of ankle if one keeps the foot in any place up to 45° plantar-flexed position—this is the **equinus position** (not deformity) of the foot, the person can actively go back to normal dorsi-flexion range. This is an anatomico-physiological phenomenon.

2. If due to paralysis of the dorsiflexors of the ankle, the foot drops in 45° plantar flexion—it is **'foot drop'**. In this condition foot can not be actively taken back to even zero position, of course, passively it can be taken back even to the maximum extent of dorsiflexion.

3. If the foot is more or less fixed in any angle up to 45° of plantar flexion from the zero position of the ankle—it is **'equinus deformity'**. In this condition, foot can not be taken back even up to zero position actively or passively. The hindfoot always remains off the ground. In such cases, where effect of equinus is produced due to spasticity of muscles such as in cerebral palsy the deformity effect can be reversed to variable extent, if the patient is taken into confidence, or the spastic muscles are relaxed by certain exercises or patient is put under anesthesia. However, if the

spasticity is allowed to continue unattended, variable fixed deformity may also develop, which must be kept in mind. These facts have to be considered while contemplating to correct the so-called equinus deformity in spastics (such as in cerebral palsy). Further, in most of the cases of equinus deformity, the culprit is tight tendoAchilles and tight plantaris accentuated by the tightness of posterior capsule of the ankle and subtalar joints. If the deformity further progresses, the magnitude of equinus deformity is exaggerated by the contracture of the capsule and ligaments on the plantar aspect of the foot, which leads to gradual development of the cavus deformity, basically in the midfoot region, and subsequently clawing of the forefoot-toes develops.

MEASUREMENT OF EQUINUS

For measurement of equinus, the patient lies supine with lower limb extended on the couch in as far as, the neutral position of the limb is possible (the mid-inguinal point, the center of centrally-placed patella, the mid-intermalleolar point and second web should be in a linear alignment). Any deviation from this alignment should be noted at the concerned level. The patient is asked to dorsiflex the foot as far as possible. The angle of limitation, viewed from outer side, to reach zero position of the ankle will be clinically-assessed as gross equinus. This should be confirmed by 'goniometer' measurement keeping its long arm over the long axis of the leg with fulcrum at a point just below the tip of lateral malleolus and short arm parallel to the 5th metatarsal (Figures 2.3A and B).

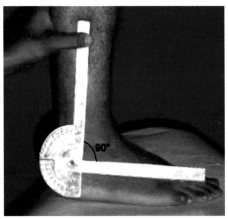

FIGURE 2.3A: Normal foot (plantigrade standing position)

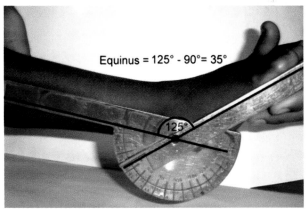

Equinus = 125° - 90° = 35°

125°

FIGURE 2.3B: Measurement of equinus by goniometer

The stretchibility of tight tendoAchilles can be assessed as follows:

From the earlier clinically-assessed position of the foot in extended knee position, it is passively dorsiflexed to as far neutral position as possible and the yield from the earlier measured equinus angle will be the possible range which can be achieved by physically stretching against the deformity. It is always better to stretch the ankle against the equinus deformity for few days to weeks prior to embarking on the surgical procedure.

CORRECTION OF EQUINUS DEFORMITY

Before contemplating to correct the equinus deformity, few questions must be answered: (1) Do all equinus deformities need correction? (2) What should be the criteria for selecting the case for correction? (3) Compensatory equinus in short limb should be left as such or corrected?

The above questions are not so easy to answer, however on over all consideration, except for the case where equinus has developed as a compensatory mechanism, other equinus deformities can be corrected on its merit.

Depending upon the age of presentation, extent of equinus, the neglect of the deformity associated with other deformities in the limb and trunk, the facilities available and expertise of surgeon, the modality of management should be selected. There is hardly any role of non-operative management in the equinus deformity. Of course, if surgery is not done (due to any cause), the shoe should be modified to accommodate and assist the equinus deformity.

Surgery has a definite role in the correction of the equinus deformity. Of course, the type of surgery will vary according to the need and extent of deformity. The basic principle of correction of equinus involves lengthening of contracted tendoAchilles tendon, which is the main culprit. There are various methods of lengthening of tendoAchilles.

1. Percutaneous subtotal tenotomy
   a. Single stab method
   b. Two stab method
2. Open procedure
   a. Open Z-lengthening of tendoAchilles
   b. Pandey's V-Y lengthening in continuity

Equinus deformity is corrected by Ilizarov method, especially, in neglected cases where correction is achieved by gradual coordinated controlled stretching of the contracted soft tissue. However, if the deformity is due to bony deformation, certain osteotomy will help in gradual stretching of the contracted soft tissue.

Most of the deformities are cosmetically unacceptable. The patient should be treated early, because more energy consumption occurs during locomotion and the potential level of activity of the patient gets gradually decelerated.

Certain deformities do develop as the compensatory mechanism to conceal, minimize or antagonize certain deficits in the body mechanism. Equinus deformity can develop as compensatory mechanism to overcome certain deficits like shortening of the limb, weakness of quadriceps muscles or even instability (to certain extent) at the knee level. Hence, a thorough clinical assessment is mandatory before contemplating the correction of equinus deformity, lest, patient will be robbed off his compensatory process.

Whatever advancements may be there in various fields of medicine, their utility can not be properly passed down to the patient unless proper selection of the patient is done. There have been tremendous advancements in the modality of investigations, however, utility of proper methodical clinical examination can not be undermined in any way while assessing a patient with deformity for proper treatment.

Clinical assessment of the deformity of foot must be done in its totality. A cursory examination of the patient as a whole and proper regional examination of spine, pelvis, hip, thigh, knee and leg must be done before embarking on the examination of foot and ankle.

In the clinical assessment of equinus, at the outset itself, it should be determined whether equinus deformity is compensatory or not. If by any means, it appears to be compensatory, the basic cause for which compensatory equinus has developed must be pin-pointed. First, determine whether contractural effect has been confined to the soft tissues alone or secondary bony and joint involvements have also occurred.

The secondary effect of equinus in different parts of foot should be assessed categorically like shape, size and position of heel, development of cavus, status of plantar ligaments, development of clawing of toes, development of callosities and fanning out of the toes.

If it is a unilateral affection, the comparative assessment with the normal foot will be more beneficial, of course, in bilateral affection separate categorical assessment is mandatory.

Exact measurement of equinus is rather difficult in terms of geometrical angulations, since the component of deformities becomes distributed in advanced cases. Initially, the fulcrum of equinus is at the ankle joint, but gradually with the advancing deformity, various grades of plantar flexion (with or without subluxation) at intertarsal and tarsometatarsal joints accentuate the equinus effect. However, a gross assessment of equinus at the ankle should be initially considered and measured to the possible extent.

INVESTIGATIONS

Basic investigations (like routine haemogram, and urine analysis) are required. Radiological evaluation is necessary to assess the deviated position and interrelationship of the bones of the foot, any associated bony or joint problems and radiological measurement of different angles. The basic X-ray view like antero-posterior view of both ankles in symmetrical position; lateral view of both ankles and feet in a symmetrical position of the foot (as far as possible); and supero-inferior (dorso-plantar) view of both feet are required (Figures 2.4A to C).

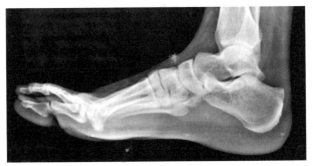

FIGURE 2.4A: Lateral view foot

For radiological measurement of equinus, true lateral view of the lower half of leg, ankle and foot is essential. The angle sustained between the long axis of the leg and long axis of the foot as viewed in lateral exposure will be the measurement of radiological angle. In this exposure itself, tibio-first metatarsal angle, tibio-calcaneal angle and calcaneometatarsal angle should be calculated. These measurements provide pre and post-treatment assessment and academic records and further help in analyzing the post-treatment position.

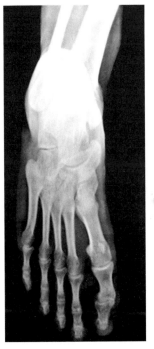 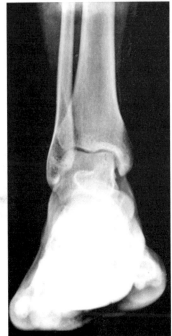

FIGURE 2.4B: Dorsoplantar supero-inferior view

FIGURE 2.4C: AP view of ankle

FIGURES 2.4A to C: Normal X-rays of foot and ankle

The main angles visible in the lateral view are tibio-first metatarsal (T.M.) angle, tibio-calcaneal (T.C.) angle and calcaneo-metatarsal (C.M.) angle in the plantigrade foot.

The tibio-first metatarsal (T.M.) angle between the axis of the tibia and the axis of the 1st metatarsal is normally 110° (Figure 2.5A).

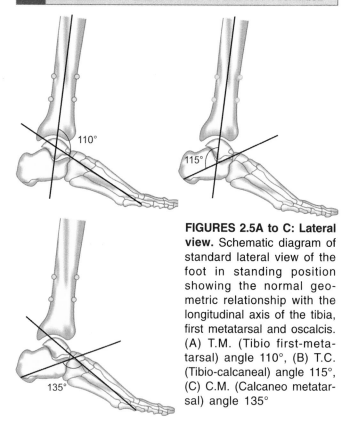

FIGURES 2.5A to C: Lateral view. Schematic diagram of standard lateral view of the foot in standing position showing the normal geometric relationship with the longitudinal axis of the tibia, first metatarsal and oscalcis. (A) T.M. (Tibio first-metatarsal) angle 110°, (B) T.C. (Tibio-calcaneal) angle 115°, (C) C.M. (Calcaneo metatarsal) angle 135°

The tibio-calcaneal (T.C.) angle formed between the axis of the tibia and the axis of the calcaneus is normally 115° (Figure 2.5B).

The calcaneo-metatarsal (C.M.) angle formed between the axis of the metatarsal and the axis of the calcaneus is normally 135° (Figure 2.5C).

The main angles visible in the dorso-plantar (supero-inferior) view are talo-first metatarsal (Ta.M.) and talo-calcaneal (Ta.C) angle (Figures 2.6A and B).

The talo-first metatarsal (Ta.M) angle between axis of talus and the axis of 1st metatarsal is normally 0° to 7°.

The talo-calcaneal (Ta.C) angle between axis of talus and axis of 1st metatarsal is normally 25° to 50°.

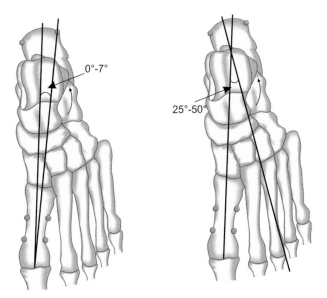

FIGURES 2.6A and B: Frontal view. Standard supero-inferior (dorso-plantar view) radiograph of foot showing talo-metatarsal (Ta.M.) normal angle 0 to 7°, talo-calcaneus (Ta.C) normal angle 25° to 50°. Like the frontal plane, deformities are visualized best in frontal view, e.g. forefoot adduction or abduction and hind foot varus and valgus

Chapter 3

TendoAchilles Lengthening

There are various methods of lengthening of tendoAchilles:

1. Percutaneous method
- i. Single stab method
- ii. Two stab method

2. Open method
- i. Z-lengthening
- ii. Pandey V–Y lengthening

PERCUTANEOUS METHOD

Single Stab Method

One fingerbreadth above the insertion of tendoAchilles, 2/3 to 3/4 of the girth of the Achilles tendon is severed by no. 15 B.P blade from anterior aspect. The surgeon's another hand holds the forefoot in maximum possible dorsiflex position of the foot from the very beginning. As the tendoAchilles gets severed the dorsiflexed position of the foot increases with stretching of the weakened tendon. This gives a ladder pattern cut of the tendon even though the position of the blade has been kept static (Figures 3.1A to I operative demonstration in a fresh cadaver for easy understanding). With further continued increase of force for dorsiflexing tendoclasis occurs which can be heard and felt. Further dorsiflexion is stopped and foot is replaced in the original equinus position with 5° more added to achieve about 2 mm overlapping of the tenotomized ends. This position is kept static for seven days. The remaining equinus deformity is corrected gradually by Ilizarov frame @ 1 mm per day from the 7th postoperative day (0.25 mm at 7 am, 11 am, 3 pm and 7pm) (the day of tenotomy should be considered as day 1).

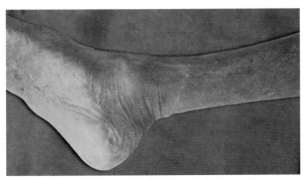

FIGURE 3.1A: Foot kept in equinus position (in a fresh cadaver)

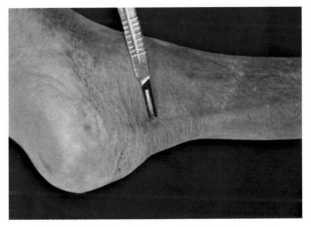

FIGURE 3.1B: Insert a no. 15 B.P blade one fingerbreadth above the insertion of tendoAchilles

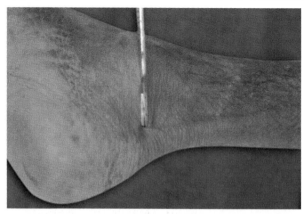

FIGURE 3.1C: While the surgeon keeps the foot tight in maximum dorsiflexed position by his left hand, the B.P blade is rotated by 90° posteriorly

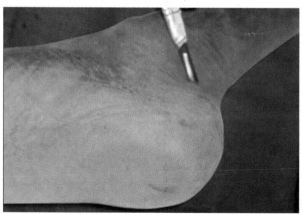

FIGURE 3.1D: While the blade remains in the same position, the tight tendoAchillis is gradually cut more or less in ladder pattern as the surgeon simultaneously keeps on increasing the passive dorsiflexion till a snapping sound of break is felt

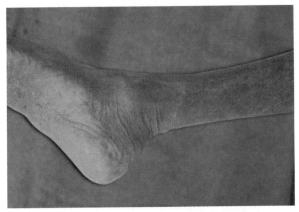

FIGURE 3.1E: The foot is further plantarflexed in its original equinus position with added 5° so that the separated tenotomized ends may overlap by 2 mm

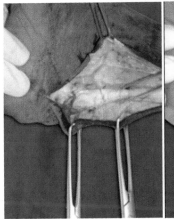
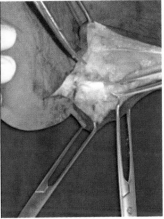

FIGURE 3.1F: Note that the tendon gets cut in ladder pattern

FIGURE 3.1G: Overlapping of tenotomized ends

The above procedure is being adopted in actual surgery for correcting the equinus deformity as shown in Figure 3.1H.

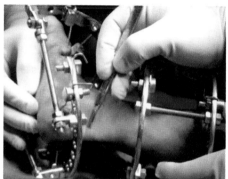

FIGURE 3.1H: All connecting threaded-rods between foot and tibia are dismantled; the percutaneous subtotal tendoAchilles tenotomy is performed; the frame is reassembled with 2 mm overriding of the tendoAchilles cut ends by increasing the original equinus by 5°

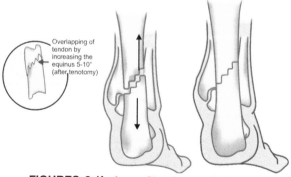

Overlapping of tendon by increasing the equinus 5-10° (after tenotomy)

FIGURES 3.1Ia to c: Showing tendoAchilles tenotomy and lengthening

FIGURES 3.1A to I: Single stab method of lengthening of tendoAchilles

Two Stab Method

One fingerbreadth above the lowest attachment of tendoAchilles, a no. 15 B.P blade is introduced at the center of the tendoAchilles parallel to its fibers. The B.P blade is turned medially cutting the medial half of the Achilles tendon. The B.P. blade is withdrawn and again inserted in the center of the Achilles tendon two fingerbreadth above the first step and the blade is turned 90° laterally cutting the lateral-half of the Achilles tendon. Then by forced dorsiflexion of the foot lengthening of tendoAchilles is achieved in continuity (medial-lateral Z lengthening in continuity). The remaining equinus deformity is corrected gradually @ 1 mm per day from the 7th postoperative day, i.e. @ 0.25 mm at 7 am, 11 am, 3 pm and 7 pm, night maneouvre is avoided so that the sleep is not disturbed (Figures 3.2A to E).

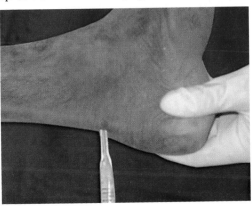

FIGURE 3.2A: A no. 15 B.P. blade is inserted in the center of the tight heel cord at one fingerbreadth above the insertion of tendoAchilles

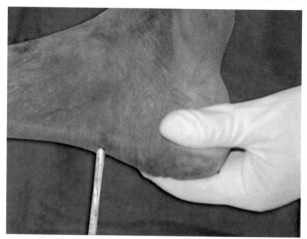

FIGURE 3.2B: The blade is turned medially by 90° which cuts the medial-half of the heel cord

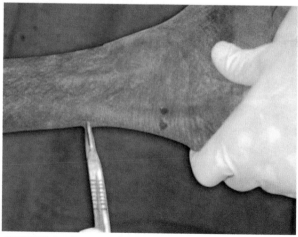

FIGURE 3.2C: Then the B.P blade is again inserted 2 fingerbreadth above the first stab in the same way

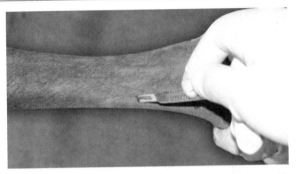

FIGURE 3.2D: Then the blade is rotated by 90° laterally which cuts the lateral-half of the heel cord at that side. The blade is withdrawn. The foot is dorsiflexed

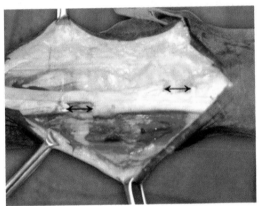

FIGURE 3.2E: The cut ends slide on each other producing the effective desired lengthening (Note that the lengthening is equal to the gap created by sliding the cut ends)

FIGURES 3.2A to E: Two stab method of lengthening of tendoAchilles as shown on fresh cadaver

The above procedure (as in Figures 3.2A to E) is being adopted in actual surgery for correcting the equinus deformity as shown in Figures 3.3A to E.

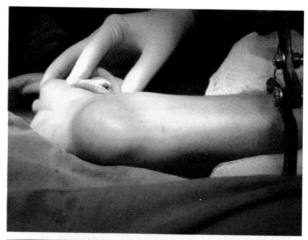

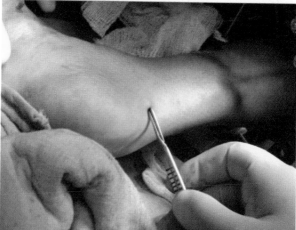

FIGURES 3.3A and B: A no. 15 B.P blade is inserted in the center of the tight heel cord at one fingerbreadth above the insertion of tendoAchilles

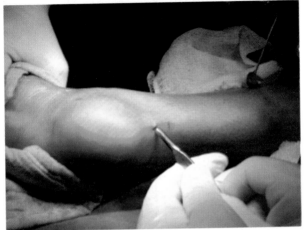

FIGURE 3.3C: The blade is turned medially by 90°
which cuts the medial-half of the heel cord

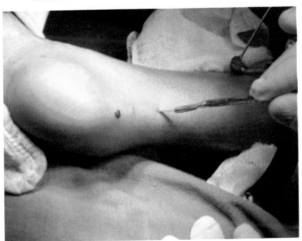

FIGURE 3.3D: The B.P. blade is again inserted two
fingerbreadth above the first stab in the same way

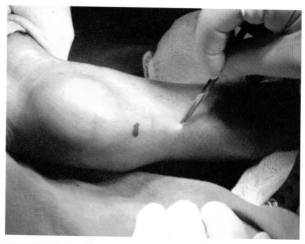

FIGURE 3.3E: Then the blade is rotated by 90° laterally which cuts the lateral-half of the heel cord at that site. The blade is withdrawn. The foot is dorsiflexed. While performing percutaneous subtotal tenotomy, the B.P. blade should be handled carefully and piercing of posterior skin must be avoided

OPEN METHOD

Z-lengthening of tendoAchilles

A vertical incision is made starting from the insertion of the tendoAchilles to the calcaneus to its musculotendinous junction parallel to the tendon on its medial side. The subcutaneous tissue is divided in the line of incision and retracted on both sides to expose the Achilles tendon covered with paratenon. After vertically diving the paratenon, the contracted tendoAchilles is cleared in its entire length and lengthened in a 'Z' fashion, the medial-half being released at its lower end from the calcaneus. The plantaris tendon is severed at its lower end. The fibroareolar tissue is cleared and the tight fibrous sheath is slit.

By dorsiflexing the foot, the desired extent of lengthening of tendoAchilles is achieved. Keeping the foot in zero position at ankle joint the medial and lateral cut ends of tendoAchilles are opposed side-to-side and stitched. Paratenon is repaired as far as possible. The wound is closed and padded plaster cast is applied from mid thigh to distal end of foot by keeping the knee and ankle at 90°.

PANDEY V-Y LENGTHENING IN CONTINUITY

It is an open procedure in which lengthening of tendinous portion of the gastroc-soleus is done at the musculotendinous tendinous junction. In this procedure a mid line incision of about 3 cm is given at the junction of lower 1/3 to upper 2/3 of the calf. The tendinous portion of the gastroc-soleus is exposed completely. While the knee is kept extended and leg elevated by about 60° from the table top, the surgeon holds the foot tightened in maximum dorsiflexed by his left hand position and by right hand only the tendinous portion of the gastroc-soleus is cut in inverted 'V' fashion. After the last few tight tendinous fibers are cut, the tendon gets lengthened and the cut ends are separated. The deeper muscular fibers also get variably stretched to provide desired lengthening of tendon. By repeated passive dorsiflexing and planterflexing of the foot the lengthening of tendon can be obviously assessed. While foot is planterflexed the cut ends of the tendon tend to come closer and after dorsiflexing they again get separated to the lengthened extent.

V-Y lengthening of tendoAchilles as shown on fresh cadaver (Figures 3.4A to D).

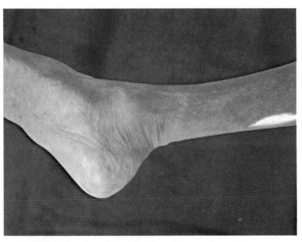

FIGURE 3.4A: A mid-line incision at the lower end of gastroc-soleus muscular belly over which the tendinous sheath is lying

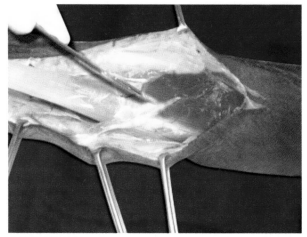

FIGURE 3.4B: The inverted 'V' cut is being performed

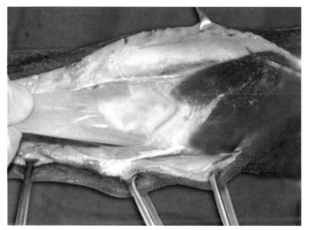

FIGURE 3.4C: Complete inverted 'V' cut has been done

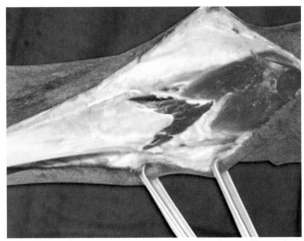

FIGURE 3.4D: With cutting of the last tendinous fibers the tendon gets lengthened while surgeon applies passive dorsiflexon force

FIGURES 3.4A to D: V-Y lengthening of tendoAchilles as shown on fresh cadaver

Chapter 4

Ilizarov: Hardware

The hardwares used in Ilizarov techniques consists of: Rings, arches, threaded rods, telescopic rods, posts (male and female), hinges (male and female), plates, bushing, thread-sockets, nuts and bolts, washer, wire fixation bolts, half pins, blocks and center sleeve for half pins, oblique support, tensioner, wrench, wires.

HALF RING

The ring is made-up of either stainless steel with a mechanical resistance greater than 90 kg/sq mm or carbon composite ring.

Available in 12 sizes, viz 80, 100, 110, 120, 130, 140, 150, 160, 180, 200, 220 and 240 mm inner diameter. Hole diameter of 8 mm with clear spacing between holes of 4 mm. Half rings are ledged at the ends to accommodate the other half right so that the assembled ring is in one plane (Figures 4.1 to 4.3).

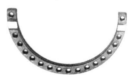

FIGURE 4.1: Steel ring

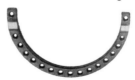

FIGURE 4.2: Carbon composite ring

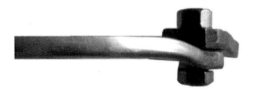

FIGURE 4.3: Connected ring

5/8 RING

Available in three sizes of inner diameter 130, 150 and 160 mm. Hole diameter and spacing are same as that of half rings (Figure 4.4). It is used near joints to facilitate movement and dressing of open wounds. It is used in combination with another full ring for reinforcement.

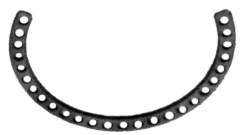

FIGURE 4.4: Ring

HALF RING WITH CURVED ENDS

5/8 rings are with outward curvature at the ends. The configuration matches the deltoid area of the shoulder and is exclusively used on shoulders (Figure 4.5).

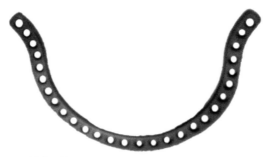

FIGURE 4.5: Half ring with curved ends

CARBON COMPOSITE FOOT RING

These rings, available in the sizes of 80, 100, 120, 140, 160 are used in hindfoot and forefoot to give better space for wires (Figure 4.6).

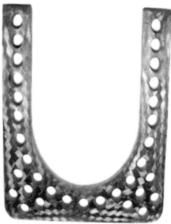

FIGURE 4.6: Carbon composite foot ring

ARCH

Russian Arch

Thicker half rings of inner diameter ranging between 80 to 260 mm are available and they are used for upper third of thigh. The staggered holes facilitate better positioning of wires (Figure 4.7).

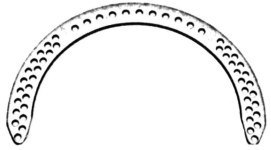

FIGURE 4.7: Russian arch

Italian Femoral Arch

These are available in section of 90° and 120°, each with small and large size. These are provided with slots and holes to secure Schanz screws/half pins and are used on upper third of thigh (Figure 4.8).

Carbon Composite Italian Femoral Arch

These are available in section of 90° and 120°, each with small and large size. These are provided with slots and holes to secure Schanz screws/half pins and are used on upper third of thigh (Figure 4.9).

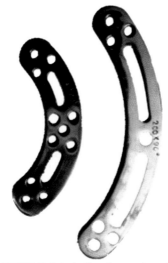

FIGURE 4.8: Italian femoral arch

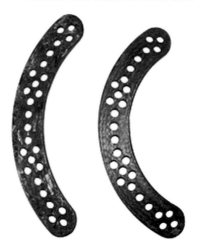

FIGURE 4.9: Carbon composite Italian femoral arch

THREADED ROD

Threaded rod is of 6 mm diameter with a thread pitch of 1 mm. These are available in lengths of 40, 60, 80, 100, 120, 150, 200, 250, 300, 350, and 400 mm to be used to interconnect rings/arches. Three connecting rods are sufficient to provide the desired mechanical strength when placed 120° apart. Since holes are engaged with other components, it is not possible to maintain 120° spacing and hence four connecting rods are used. Threaded rods can withstand high axial loading but with increased length their stability to resist bending reduces. It is advisable to keep the length of connecting rods not greater than that of the diameter of the rings (Figure 4.10).

FIGURE 4.10: Threaded rod

SLOTTED CANNULATED ROD

Some short threaded rods are grooved at one end in which a wire can be secured with two nuts to provide traction (Figure 4.11).

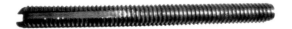

FIGURE 4.11: Slotted cannulated rod

PARTIAL THREADED ROD

These are available in the sizes of 130, 170 and 210 mm. The central portion is not threaded to prevent damage by locking nuts when used in telescopic rods (Figure 4.12).

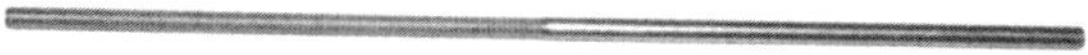

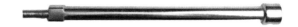

FIGURE 4.12: Partial threaded rod

TELESCOPIC ROD

It is a long hollow tube with its inner diameter larger than the outer diameter of any threaded rod. It is used to increase frame rigidity when connecting rings/arches are greater than 150 mm apart. The telescopic rod has a threaded stud at one end and a perpendicular locking bolt at the other end to hold the threaded rod. These are available in 100, 150, 200, 250, 350 and 400 mm lengths (Figure 4.13).

FIGURE 4.13: Telescopic rod

GRADUATED TELESCOPIC ROD

These are available in the sizes of 60, 100, 150, 200 and 250 mm, these rods are used in lengthening and providing direct measurement (Figure 4.14).

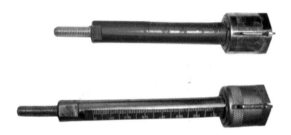

FIGURE 4.14: Graduate telescopic rod

POST

Post is a short plate with 2 to 4 smooth holes of 7 mm diameter and is used as an auxiliary support element for fixing wires/rods/plates at any angle to the main support. They can also be used as locked/mobile joints that can be assembled into multiplanar hinges (Figure 4.15).

Posts may be male or female. Male posts are 28, 38 or 48 mm long with 2, 3 and 4 holes respectively. Female posts are 30, 40 or 50 mm long with 2, 3 and 4 holes respectively.

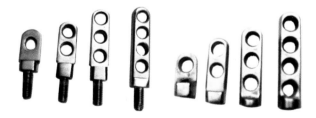

FIGURE 4.15: Post

HINGES

Hinge Female Standard and Low profile (Figure 4.16)

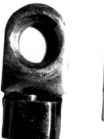

FIGURE 4.16: Hinge female
(standard and low profile)

These have a supporting base with two flat surfaces for matching standard 10 mm wrench. It has only one hole which is 4 mm thick at base. Low profile half hinges of 30 mm height are also used in multiple planes (hinges have flanges on one side).

CONSTRUCTION OF HINGE (Figure 4.17)

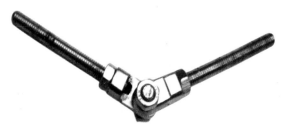

FIGURE 4.17: Constructed hinge

HINGE MALE STANDARD AND LOW PROFILE (FIGURE 4.18)

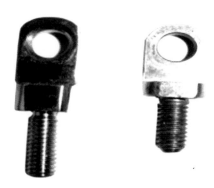

FIGURE 4.18: Male components for hinge

HINGE-90° STANDARD AND 90° LOW PROFILE (FIGURE 4.19)

In 90° hinges two flanges are positioned at right angles to the long axis and can be used as a middle component of a two-axis hinge (Figure 4.19).

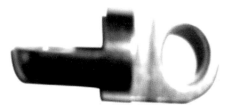

FIGURE 4.19: Hinge-90° standard

CONNECTING PLATE

Plates are used as connecting elements for connecting rings of various diameters. They are also used for various combinations in frame structure.

Plates may be straight, curved or twisted. They are all 5 mm thick, 14 mm wide and with perforated holes of 7 mm diameter.

Straight plates may be of the following types:

a. Short connection plates
b. Long connection plates
c. Connecting plates with threaded ends

Short Connecting Plate

Short connecting plates are available in 9 sizes with 2 to 10 holes. Most commonly used are 2 and 3 hole plates for extension of the main frame (Figure 4.20).

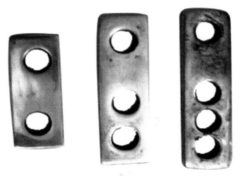

FIGURE 4.20: Short connecting plate

Long Connecting Plate

Long connecting plates are used in place of middle rings in cases of extensive soft tissue damage. Large frames can be reinforced by these plates and can also be used for translational and pivotal movements of the middle ring. They are of 155, 235 and 335 mm lengths with 8, 12 and 17 holes respectively (Figure 4.21).

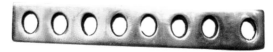

FIGURE 4.21: Long connecting plate

Connecting Plate with Threaded End

Connecting plate with threaded ends are of 135, 175, 215 and 255 mm lengths with 5, 9 and 11 holes respectively. These are used as long supporting plates and for fabrication of various configurations (Figure 4.22).

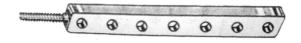

FIGURE 4.22: Connecting plate with threaded end

TWISTED PLATE

Twisted plate is used to connect long connecting plates to the frame. These plates are used to connect between holes of vertical and horizontal planes. They are of 45, 65 and 85 mm lengths with 2, 3 and 4 holes respectively (Figure 4.23).

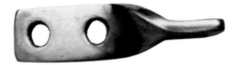

FIGURE 4.23: Twisted plate

CURVED PLATE

These are used as extension to half ring arch for accommodating K-wires. They are to be secured by a threaded rod to the adjacent ring or reinforced with an additional short plate (Figure 4.24).

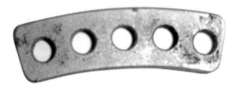

FIGURE 4.24: Curved plate

BUSHING

The bushing is of two sizes (12 mm and 24 mm) with one and two perpendicular holes. It is short 12 mm cylinder with a smooth unthreaded apperture (7 mm in diameter). It is 1 mm wider than threaded rod. It moves smoothly over the threaded rod. It is also used as spacer (Figure 4.25).

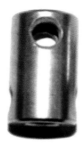

FIGURE 4.25: Bushings

THREADED SOCKET

These are of 20 and 40 mm length with external diameter of 10 mm. Both ends are threaded to accommodate bolts/ threaded rods. Two perpendicular threaded holes are provided at the center on either side to connect bolts/ rods as extension of threaded rods. These are used to connect half or 5/8 ring to the adjacent full ring for which at least three threaded sockets are used. They are also used to interconnect two full rings for reinforcing where four threaded sockets are used (Figure 4.26).

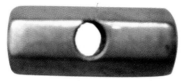

FIGURE 4.26: Threaded socket

CONNECTING BOLT

It is available in standard sizes of 10, 16, 20, and 30 mm and 4 mm thickness (Figure 4.27).

- 10 mm bolts are used only for securing threaded rods and pins through apperture of sockets, bushings and telescopic rods. It is also used for connecting threaded sockets and bushings to rings/connecting plates.
- 16 mm bolts are the most commonly used connecting bolts since the thickness of the main components vary between 4 and 5 mm and the thickness of the nuts 5 mm.
- 20 mm bolts are used to connect female hinges.
- 30 mm bolts are used to connect 3 or more parts. They can also be used at places to bridge the distance from the rings to pins/wires conveniently.

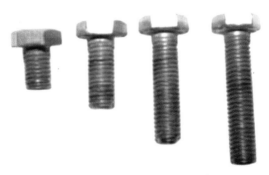

FIGURE 4.27: Connecting bolts

NUT

Nut is available in thickness of 3, 5 and 6 mm.

- Three mm nuts are used only as locking nuts on hinges.
- Five mm nuts are used for stabilizing all forms of frame construction.
- Six mm nuts are to be used on connecting rods where compression/distraction is required.

These are used at hinges to have controlled motion (Figure 4.28).

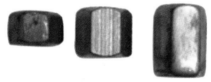

FIGURE 4.28: Nuts

NYLON INSERT NUT

Nylon insert nut is used in hinges to perform controlled motion (Figure 4.29).

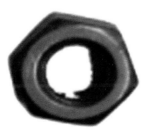

FIGURE 4.29: Nylon insert nut

QUADRANGULAR SQUARE HEAD NUT

Quadrangular square head nut is 10 mm long and have a quadrangular head. The head is marked numerically from 1 to 4 or dotted to facilitate rate of lengthening/compression (Figure 4.30).

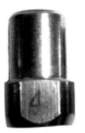
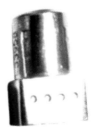

FIGURE 4.30: Quadrangular square head nut

WASHER

Washer is used to fill the space, these are of various types.

Spacing Washer

Size 1.5, 2.0 mm (Figure 4.31)

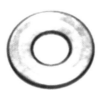
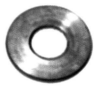

FIGURE 4.31: Spacing washer

Split Locking Washer

Size 2.0 mm (Figure 4.32)

FIGURE 4.32: Split locking washer

Flat-Sided Washer

Size 2.0 mm
Size 4.0 mm (Figure 4.33)

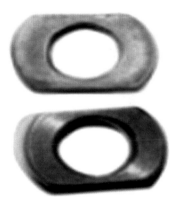

FIGURE 4.33: Flat-sided washer

Slotted Washer

Size 4.0 mm (Figure 4.34)

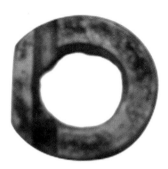

FIGURE 4.34: Slotted washer

CONICAL WASHER COUPLE (Figure 4.35)

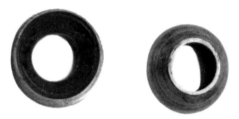

FIGURE 4.35: Conical wahser couple

WIRE FIXATION BOLT

Wire fixation bolt is used to secure the wires and can be either cannulated or slotted. These are of 6 mm threaded diameter, 18 mm length and a bolt head thickness of 6 mm. The bolt heads are either hexagonal or with two flat and rounded surfaces. Cannulated bolts have a 2 mm hole while slotted bolts have an oblique groove on the under face of the bolt head. The bolt head being double in thickness to that of a regular bolt head, it facilitates turning when the adjacent holes are occupied by other nuts/bolts (Figure 4.36).

A special cannulated bolt is also available with a head thickness of 11 mm. It has a 6 mm diameter threaded hole at the center of the head top, which allows introduction of bolts/rods when needed under special circumstances.

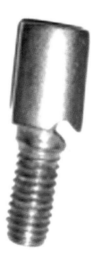

FIGURE 4.36: Wire fixation bolt

WIRE FIXATION CANNULATED BOLT

Cannulated bolts are preferred for 1.5 mm wires and slotted bolts for 1.8 mm wires. For optimal tightening, it is advisable to use 5 mm nuts with wire fixation bolts. Because of metal fatigue, wire fixation bolts should never be reused (Figure 4.37).

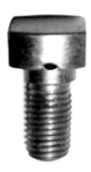

FIGURE 4.37: Wire fixation cannulated bolt

WIRE FIXATION BOLT WITH THREADED SOCKET

The wire fixation bolt with threaded socket has dual function (Figure 4.38) for fixation of wire and connecting threaded rod.

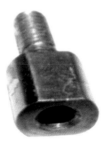

FIGURE 4.38: Wire fixation bolt with threaded socket

BLOCK FOR HALF PIN

Size 1,2,3,4, and 5 holes (Figure 4.39)

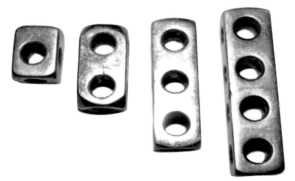

FIGURE 4.39: Block for half pin

BLOCK FOR HALF PIN FOR CENTER SLEEVE

Size 1,2,3,4, and 5 holes (Figure 4.40)

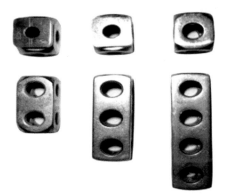

FIGURE 4.40: Block for half pin for center sleeve

CENTER SLEEVE FOR BLOCK FOR HALF PIN (Figure 4.41)

FIGURE 4.41: Center sleeve for block for half pin

BOX WRENCH FOR BOLT

Box wrench is used to tight and loosen the nut (Figure 4.42).

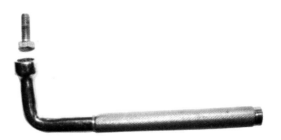

FIGURE 4.42: Box wrench for bolt

OBLIQUE SUPPORT

Oblique support is used to connect Italian arch with ring (Figure 4.43).

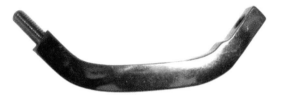

FIGURE 4.43: Oblique support

SOCKET WRENCH FOR WIRE FIXATION BOLT (Figure 4.44)

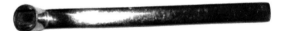

FIGURE 4.44: Socket wrench for wire fixation bolt

COMBINATION WRENCH (10 MM) (Figure 4.45)

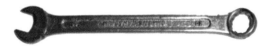

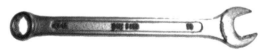

FIGURE 4.45: Combination wrench (10 mm)

WIRE TENSIONER-MECHANICAL (Figure 4.46)

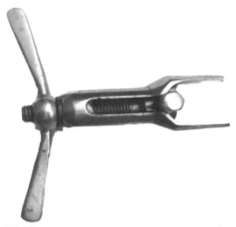

FIGURE 4.46: Wire tensioner-mechanical

WIRE TENSIONER DIRECT MEASURING (Figure 4.47)

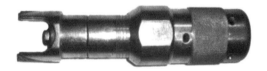

FIGURE 4.47: Wire tensioner direct measuring

OSTEOTOME AND KEY

Size 3, 5, 7 and 9 mm (Figure 4.48).

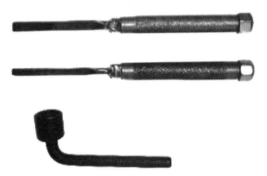

FIGURE 4.48: Osteotome and key

CORTICOTOME

Size 3,5,7 and 9 mm (Figure 4.49).

FIGURE 4.49: Corticotome

IMPLANTS

Wires

The Bayonet point (Figures 4.50A and B): It is used mainly for diaphysis of long bones as it has greater penetrating power. The advantage of bayonet point is that it causes less heating effect of bones and soft tissues. It produces hole of a diameter slightly larger than that of wire thus causing less friction.

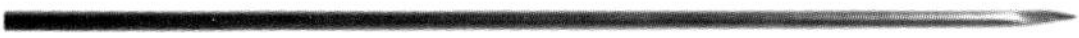

FIGURE 4.50A: Bayonet point-cortical 1.5 mm x 300 mm
It is used in the diaphysis of forearm and foot bones

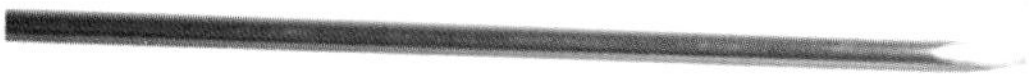

FIGURE 4.50B: Bayonet point—cortical 1.8 mm x 370 mm
It is used in the diaphysis of tibia and femur

The Trocar point (Figures 4.50C and D): Trocar point is used in the metaepiphyseal regions of bones because it has less penetrating power. It produces the hole of exactly the same diameter as of the wire. The advantage of trocar point is that it has greater hold in the bones.

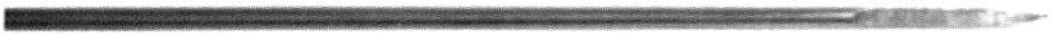

FIGURE 4.50C: Trocar point—cancellous 1.5 mm x 300 mm
It is used in the metaepiphyseal region of forearm bone

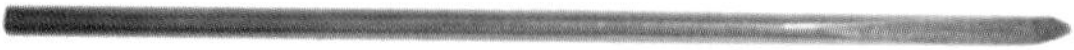

FIGURE 4.50D: Trocar point—cancellous 1.8 mm x 370 mm
It is used in the metaepiphyseal region of tibia and femur

Olive or Stopper Wire (Figures 4.50E and F): The olive wire is used to achieve and maintain the position of principle fragment after fracture. It is also used to hold the fragment during correction of deformities.

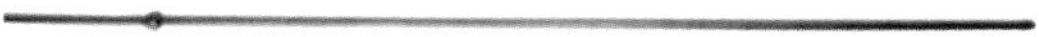

FIGURE 4.50E: With stopper (Bayonet point) 1.5 x 300 mm

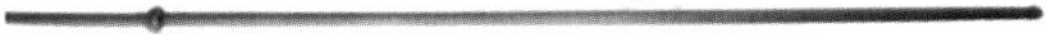

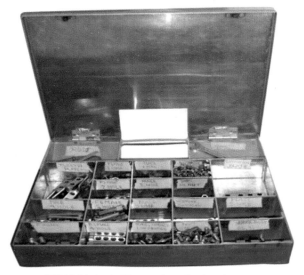

FIGURE 4.50F: With stopper (Bayonet point) 1.8 x 400 mm

ILIZAROV BOX FOR HARDWARE (FIGURE 4.51)

FIGURE 4.51: Ilizarov box for hardware

Chapter 5

Ilizarov: Basic Principles

We have earlier noted that there are several methods of managing these deformities, but in this monograph our main aim is to highlight the use of Ilizarov technique for correcting the equinus deformity of the foot and ankle.

There are three broad aspects of Ilizarov technique in correcting the deformity—

1. The patient and attendants must be clearly explained about the technique, the hardware and the need of their co-operation throughout the treatment. The ultimate result depends more on the patient and attendant's acceptance and continued co-operation.

2. Selection of the rings and pins and other fixative adjuncts and instruments.

3. A proper rehearsal of constructing the frames and placement of frames on the extremity should be done prior to actual procedure.

SELECTION OF POINTS FOR PASSING K-WIRES:

The selection of points for passing K-wires should be considered broadly in two sets of configuration:

1. First configuration is indicated where lengthening of tibia is required along with correction of deformity. Here three sets of cross-wires are passed in the leg bones—the proximal, middle and distal.

2. The second configuration is indicated where only correction of deformity is required. Here two sets of

wires are passed at about the junction of proximal to the middle-third and middle to the distal-third.

Points for passing K- wires in Leg

Proximal Tibial Wires

In the proximal set, the first wire (1.8 mm) enters through the center of the head of fibula with an inclination aiming parallel to knee joint line and to emerge at a point just posterior to the vertical line coming from the medial border of patella. The second wire enters on the anterolateral surface of upper end of tibia just behind and about 5 mm (note that the thickness of ring – 4 mm) below the point created by the horizontal line of the head of fibula and vertical line coming down from lateral border of patella with an inclination of the wire aiming to emerge at same level just anterior to the medial border (Figure 5.1). In cases of tibial lengthening a 3rd wire may also be passed from the lateral side anterior to the head of fibula aiming to emerge on medial side at the same level.

Middle Tibial Wires

Two K-wires (1.8 mm) are inserted at the junction of upper and middle-third of tibia. The first wire is inserted at about one fingerbreadth lateral and behind the shin of tibia with an inclination of the wire aiming to emerge at the same level just anterior to the medial border. Second wire is inserted about one fingerbreadth anterior to the palpable

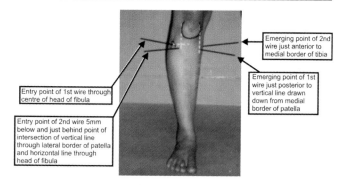

FIGURE 5.1: Proximal tibial wires Note: In case of carbon ring both the wires should be 7 mm apart

anterior border of fibula at a point about 5 mm (thickness of ring 4 mm) below the level of first wire and with an inclination anteriorly aiming the wire to emerge about one fingerbreadth posteromedial to shin of tibia at about the same level (Figure 5.2).

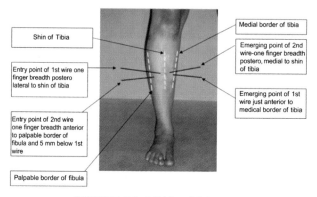

FIGURE 5.2: Middle tibial wires

Distal Tibial Wires

Two K-wires (1.8 mm diameter) are inserted at the junction of distal and middle-third of tibia. The first wire of this set is inserted through fibula and passed through the tibia with an inclination aiming the wire to emerge one fingerbreadth posteromedial to the shin of tibia (Figure 5.3). The point of selection for inserting the second wire should be done cautiously. The space between the anterior border of tibia and fibula is divided into three equal zones. The anterior zone contains neurovascular structures and tendons. The middle zone is more or less safe containing mostly the muscular part. At about 5 mm (note that the thickness of ring 4 mm) below the level of the first wire, the second wire is inserted through the safe corridor of middle zone into the tibia with an inclination to emerge just anterior to the medial border of tibia. (Figure 5.4). One should be careful to avoid piercing the great saphenous vein which crosses the medial border of tibia about 5 fingerbreadth above medial malleolus in anteroposterior direction (Figures 5.5 to 5.7).

Placement of Half Pin / Schanz Screw

The K-wire passes through muscles hence there are possibilities of certain complications including pain, and neurovascular injuries. Reduction in number of wires decreases the problems of pain and neurovascular injuries but it can reduce the strength and stability of the configuration. Hybrid (wire and half-pins) Ilizarov fixators

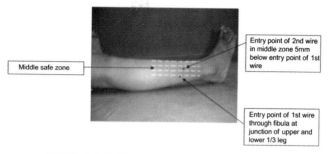

Middle safe zone

Entry point of 2nd wire in middle zone 5mm below entry point of 1st wire

Entry point of 1st wire through fibula at junction of upper and lower 1/3 leg

FIGURE 5.3: Entry point of distal tibial wires

Exit point of 1st wire one finger breadth posteromedial to shin of tibia

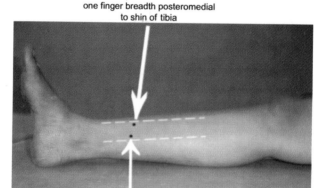

Exit of 2nd wire just anterior to medial border of tibia

FIGURE 5.4: Exit point of 1st and 2nd wire

and half-pin fixators are also being used in an attempt to alleviate these problems by minimal transfixation of the surrounding soft tissues and cautious insertion of wires through anatomically safe zones (Fleming et al and Green 1992).

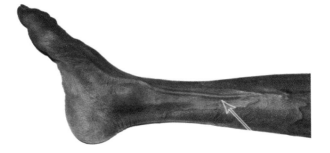

FIGURE 5.5: Course of great saphenous vein

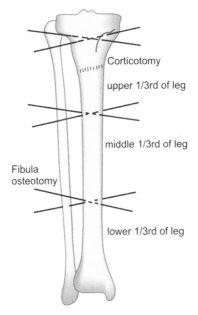

FIGURE 5.6: Position of wires for proximal, middle and
distal tibial rings

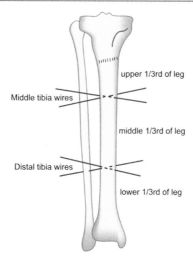

upper 1/3rd of leg

Middle tibia wires

middle 1/3rd of leg

Distal tibia wires

lower 1/3rd of leg

FIGURE 5.7: Position of wires for middle and distal tibial rings

To avoid piercing through muscles as far as possible, the second wire in proximal and distal sets and both wires of middle set can be replaced by 5 mm Schanz screw which enters from one cortex and just pierces the opposite cortex to secure firm fixation. However, in children and adolescents Schanz screw should be avoided where it has to pass through growth plate.

However, there is possibility of varied loosening of the Schanz screw, which is passed through metaphyseal region. It has to be noted that in proximal set, two 5 mm Schanz screws are passed one from either side more or less at the point of entrance and emergence of second wire, of course some adjustment of the level of screws is needed to avoid the end–on obstruction of the screws, (usually screws should be avoided in metaphysis). It is important to note that in proximal and distal sets, four point fixations are mandatory. However, when Schanz screws are used even less than 4-point purchase can provide firmness (since screw has greater holding capacity than round K-wire). In the middle set where 5 mm Schanz screws can replace one or even both the wires, the screw should remain localized in between the shin and medial border of tibia, of course with the provision of getting the maximum angle between them. In distal set as well, the precaution should be taken to pass the 5 mm Schanz screw (which can replace only one wire) from one cortex to other cortex in between the shin and medial border of tibia with maximum angulation (Figure 5.8).

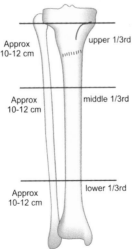

FIGURE 5.8: Position of Schanz screws for proximal, middle and distal tibial rings

Proximal Tibial Schanz Screw

To facilitate the proper positioning of the proximal ring it is observed that one **reference** wire should be passed first from the anterolateral region of the flare of lateral condyle of tibia one fingerbreadth in front and one fingerbreadth above the head of fibula parallel to knee joint—(approx 14 mm below the subchondral line of joint to avoid articular penetration) to emerge on the same level through the flare of medial condyle of tibia then second K-wire is passed from the center of the head of fibula with an inclination to emerge at a point just posterior to the vertical line dropping from the medial border of patella.

After that one Schanz screw is passed through the anterolateral surface of upper end of tibia from a point about 12 mm below the reference wire on the vertical line drawn from the lateral border of patella. The screw goes with an inclination to engage the thicker cortex just behind the medial border (Figure 5.9A).

Alternatively, another configuration can be created by using reference wire, first Schanz screw (as passed in earlier configuration) and second Schanz screw from the antero-medial aspect of upper end of tibia is threaded over the second K-wire which were passed from the center of the head of fibula. Practically, a cannulated drill (started from the medial side) is used over the medial projecting end of the K-wire to facilitate the passing of second Schanz screw, which ends by just passing through the lateral cortex of tibia and engaging into the head of fibula (Figure 5.9B).

Further modification can be done to avoid passing of K-wire or Schanz screw in the head of fibula by passing a syndosmotic screw (or cancellous screw) from the fibular head to the upper end of tibia, this has the advantage of checking the upper end of fibula from being disturbed in the process of lengthening maneuver in the apparatus.

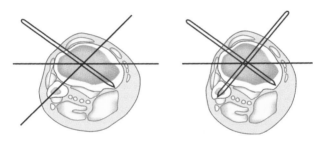

A   **B**
FIGURES 5.9A and B: Placement of proximal Schanz screws

Middle Tibial Schanz Screw

In the middle set either one K-wire and one screw is passed (Figure 5.10A) or two Schanz screws replace the K-wire (Figure 5.10B).

Distal Tibial Schanz Screw

The first wire of this set is inserted through fibula and passed through tibia with an inclination aiming the wire

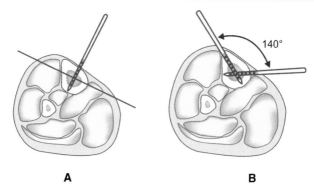

A **B**

FIGURES 5.10A and B: Placement of middle tibial Schanz screws. A. One K-wire is passed one fingerbreadth lateral and posterior to the shin of tibia, which emerges anterior to the medial border of tibia; and one Schanz screw is passed from the medial surface of tibia. B. First Schanz screw is passed from medial border of tibia and another Schanz screw from the shin of tibia

to emerge one fingerbreadth postero-medial to the shin of tibia. First Schanz screw is fixed from medial border of tibia and the second Schanz screw from medial surface of tibia making maximum angle at a distance from first screw with the help of three to four hole block for half pin (Figure 5.11).

Points of Passing Wires in Foot

Usually, three sets of two wires are required to be passed in the foot. One set (1.8 mm) passes through the calcaneum, second set (1.5 mm) through the mid-tarsal region and third set (1.5 mm) through more or less distal

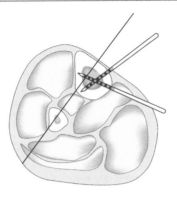

FIGURE 5.11: Placement of Schanz screw in
lower-third of tibia

end of metatarsals just proximal to the metatarsal head.
Wires in the foot are not tensioned.

Calcaneal Wires

Medial approach: Though it appears handy to insert the
K-wire from lateral side of calcaneus but several times
there remains the possibility of emerging the K-wire
variably stray in relation to the desired exit point and in
such situation there is risk of damage of neurovascular
bundle and to avoid this risk the K-wires can also be passed
from medial side. The pulsation of posterior tibial artery
should be felt and posterior tibial nerve can also be
palpated. One and a half fingerbreadth behind the
posterior tibial artery pulsation / posterier tibial nerve
palpation will be the safe zone on the medial surface of

calcaneus which comes about two and a half to three fingerbreadth behind the posterior border of posterior malleolus (the feeling of pulsation of tibialis posterior will be a more safeguard to avoid the catastrophe). On this surface the first K-wire is inserted at one fingerbreadth above the under surface of calcaneus and one fingerbreadth in front of insertion of tendoAchilles. The wire is advanced anterolaterally at an inclination of 30°. The second wire is inserted at a point 1cm anterior to the first point and 1cm above the inferior surface of calcaneus. The wire is advanced laterally to emerge 1cm above the inferior surface and 1cm distal to attachment of tendoAchilles. In this configuration the angles sustained between the two wires are more or less 30° (Figures 5.12 and 5.14).

Lateral approach: In the calcaneus the first wire is inserted on the outer surface of calcaneus about 1 cm above its inferior surface and 1 cm distal to the attachment of tendoAchilles. The wire is advanced with an inclination anteromedially aiming to emerge on the medial surface of the calcaneus two fingerbreadth below the medial malleolus (to avoid any damage to neurovascular bundle). The second wire is inserted one fingerbreadth distal to the entry point of the first wire and is advanced obliquely posteromedially to emerge about one fingerbreadth behind the first wire in the same level. In this configuration the angles sustained between the two wires are more or less 30° (Figures 5.13 and 5.14).

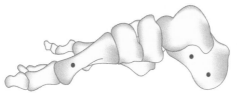

FIGURE 5.12: Wire position in calcaneus and metatarsals

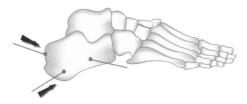

FIGURE 5.13: Wires in calcaneus

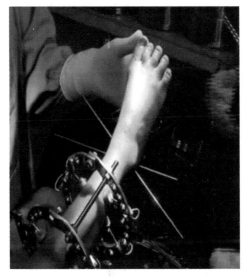

FIGURE 5.14: Wires in calcaneus

Position of Wires in Midtarsal Region

If cavus is associated with equinus deformity, two additional K-wire of 1.5 mm are required to correct such deformity, one K-wire is passed on the medial surface just below the nevicular tuberosity to emerge at the summit of the cavus and other wire is initiated at the center of outer surface of cuboid and is passed again aiming to emerge in the summit of the cavus and both the K-wires to make the an angle of 30° between them. Wires are not tensioned (Figure 5.15).

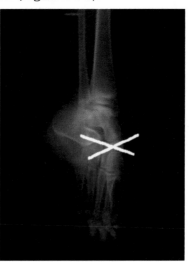

FIGURE 5.15: Position of K-wire in midtarsal region

Wires at the Base of Metatarsal Head

In the distal configuration, the first wire is inserted from the outer side through the distal part of the fifth metatarsal between the head and neck and is advanced obliquely piercing the fifth, fourth and third metatarsal just proximal to their heads to emerge on the surface on the dorsum of the foot. The second wire is inserted on the medial surface in the distal first metatarsal just proximal to its head and advances obliquely to emerge on the dorsum of foot after piercing through second metatarsal. Figures 5.16 A to C)

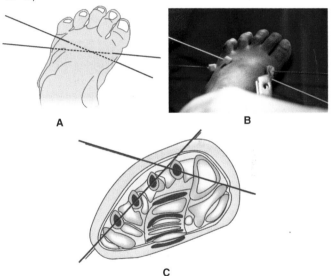

A   B

C

FIGURES 5.16A to C: Position of K-wires in standard approach

To avoid interfering with the transverse metatarsal arch a modified approach (Figures 5.16A to C) is being practised where the first wire is inserted just distal to the neck of fifth metatarsal at the outer surface and is advanced obliquely to pierce the first metatarsal and ultimately to emerge anteromedially on the medial surface of the first ray. It also pierces the fourth metatarsal. The second wire is inserted from the dorsal surface piercing proximal to the head of the third metatarsal and is advanced piercing the second and first metatarsal ultimately emerging on the medial surface of the foot (Figures 5.17A to C).

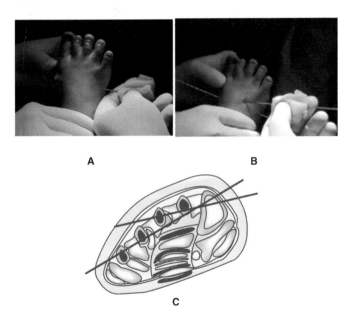

A   B

C

FIGURES 5.17A to C: Position of K-wires in the forefoot (modified approach). A. Wire position in the fifth, fourth and first metatarsals. B. Wire position in the third, second and first metatarsals. C. Transverse section of metatarsal

SIZE OF THE RINGS

The size of the ring should allow clearance at least of two fingerbreadth at the maximum girth of the limb. All the three rings should be of the same size.

POSITION OF RINGS

Proximal Tibial Ring

This ring is to be used only when simultaneous lengthening is being contemplated. A full ring is placed at the level of the head of fibula. (Figures 5.18 A and B)

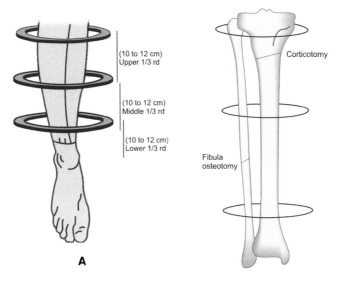

A

FIGURES 5.18A and B: Position of rings in tibial lengthening

Middle Tibial Ring

A full ring is placed approximately at the junction of upper third to middle third of the leg (Figure 5.19).

Distal Tibial Ring

A full ring is placed about 10-12 cm above the ankle joint, i.e. at about the junction of lower-third and middle third of leg (Figure 5.19).

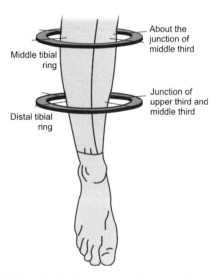

Middle tibial ring

About the junction of middle third

Distal tibial ring

Junction of upper third and middle third

FIGURE 5.19: Position of middle and distal ring

Half Calcaneal Ring

The half calcaneal ring should be placed behind and parallel to plantar surface of heel, which will be more or less horizontal when the patient stands, however, in cases of varus or valgus deformity the inclination of the ring will be according to the concerned deformity (and will not be horizontal) (Figure 5.20).

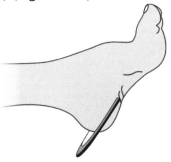

FIGURE 5.20: Placement of the ring in calcaneus

Half Forefoot Ring

In the forefoot the half ring is placed proximal to the head of metatarsals and the ring should be perpendicular to the head of metatarsals (Figure 5.21).

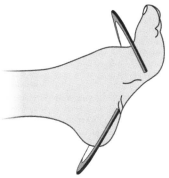

FIGURE 5.21: Placement of rings in calcaneus and forefoot

Full Ring at Forefoot

If the equinus deformity is associated with the cavus foot, a full ring should be placed around the forefoot. (Figure 5.22).

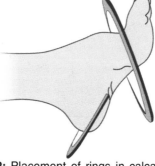

FIGURE 5.22: Placement of rings in calcaneus and forefoot

Half Ring in Mid-Foot

A half ring is also needed in the mid-foot when equinus is associated with cavus deformity (Figure 5.23).

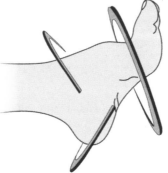

FIGURE 5.23: Placement of half ring in mid-foot region

Full Ring in Mid-Foot

A half ring is also needed in the mid-foot when equinus is associated with severe equinocavus deformity (Figure 5.24).

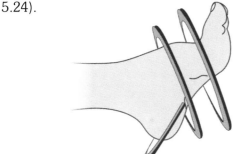

FIGURE 5.24: Placement of full ring in mid-foot region

CONSTRUCTION OF THE FRAME

Placement of Pre-constructed Frames (Leg and Foot)

Pre-construction of frame is necessary to save time during the surgery. We usually make plaster mould of deformed leg and foot and pre-constructed frame is tried over it before mounting it on the patient's leg.

The frame construction will be different in both the situations, i.e. first for correcting of equinus deformity alone and second for correcting the equinus deformity along with lengthening of short leg (Figures 5.25A and B).

For correcting equinus deformity alone proximal ring is not required, the middle and the distal ring serves the purpose (Figure 5.26).

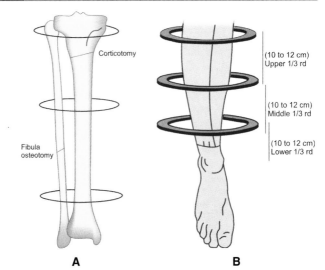

FIGURES 5.25A and B: Position of rings for tibial
lengthening

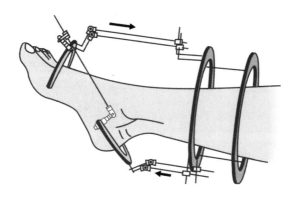

FIGURE 5.26: Complete frame assembly with two anterior
and two posterior threaded rods

EQUINUS WITH SHORT LEG

When shortening is associated with equinus deformity the correction of equinus deformity and lengthening of tibia is done simultaneously. The fibula osteotomy is done before applying the frame, followed by tibial corticotomy for lengthening of the tibia.

Osteotomy of Fibula

Osteotomy of fibula is performed above the junction of middle-third and lower-third of fibula. In poliomyelitis, level of osteotomy is at the mid-shaft of fibula because of muscle wasting.

One to two cm longitudinal incision is given anteriorly over fibula and 10 to 15 mm osteotome is inserted in longitudinal direction to feel the fibula, and then osteotome is rotated by 90° with 10 to 15° of obliquity (Figures 5.27A to C).

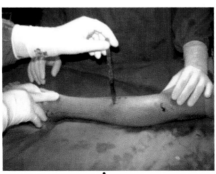

A

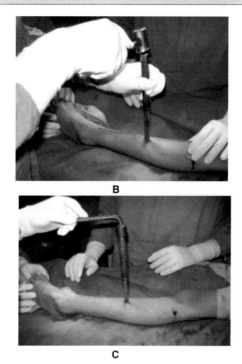

FIGURES 5.27A to C: Fibula osteotomy A. Insertion of knife; B. Insertion of osteotome; C. Rotation of osteotome 90°

Corticotomy of Tibia

Threaded rods of proximal and middle rings of tibia are dismantled and 10 to 15 mm longitudinal incision is given 1 cm below and lateral to tibial tuberosity. Five to ten mm osteotome is inserted from lateral side up to the bone longitudinally. Osteotome is then rotated 90° and corticotomy is performed.

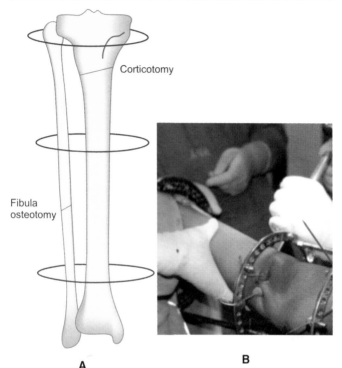

FIGURES 5.28A and B: Corticotomy of tibia

The method of passing the wires, placing the rings, connecting the wires to the rings, connecting the rods, tensioning the wires, fibula osteotomy, corticotomy of tibia (Figrues 5.28A and B) and final adjustment of the frame for the correction of shortening associated with equinus deformity have been detailed in step by step on the (Figures 6.32A-AQ).

POSTOPERATIVE CORRECTION

The correction starts from the 7th postoperative day (the day of surgery is considered as day one). Before starting correction; mathematical calculation has to be done for soft tissue distraction. Distraction of soft tissues can be performed up to 3 mm. The equinus is corrected by tightening of anterior threaded rods and loosening of posterior threaded rods.

This process of loosening and tightening of threaded rods should be performed four times a day (@ 0.25 mm), at 7 am, 11 am, 3 pm and 7 pm so that the patient's sleep is not disturbed at night. At the time of correction, all hinges should be loosened and after correction all the hinges should be tightened otherwise frame will be unstable and regeneration of tendoAchilles may be affected, but if the tenotomy of tendoAchilles is not done, only soft tissue distraction is done then hinges remain fixed with the nylon nuts, which provides controlled smooth motion. After achieving 10° to 15° of equinus correction the position of proximal hinges should be adjusted accordingly.

The frame should be retained for a minimum period of six weeks after full correction or equal to the time consumed in achieving the correction except for bone lengthening.

Chapter 6

Correction for Equinus Deformity

Equinus deformity denotes foot fixed in plantar flexed position. Cavus refers to the increased height of the vault of the foot. Usually the deformity develops first in sagittal, followed by horizontal and lastly in the frontal plane. Deformities are corrected in reverse direction, i.e. firstly in frontal, then in horizontal and lastly in sagittal plane. Deformity of each segment will be considered separately as deformities develop gradually.

SAGITTAL PLANE DEFORMITY

In sagittal plane, the axis of rotation passes through ankle joint. The motions in sagittal plane are dorsiflexion and plantar flexion. Moreover, the deformities occur mainly at the ankle joint but may also occur at midtarsal joints after the full range of plantar flexion is exhausted at the ankle level. Usually dorsiflexion and plantar flexion motion take place at ankle joint but the plantar flexion motion also takes place in midtarsal joint as may be noticed in a ballet dancer's foot where the angle may be up to 180° (Figure 6.1).

EQUINUS DEFORMITY

Anatomically, the normal range of dorsiflexion is upto 20° and plantar flexion at ankle joint is up to 45° to 50° (Figure 6.2).

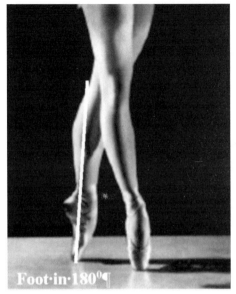

FIGURE 6.1: A ballet dancer's feet (showing angle 180°)

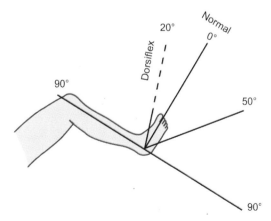

FIGURE 6.2: Range of motion at ankle joint (plantar flexion)

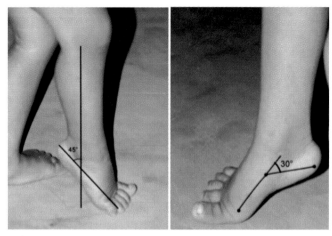

FIGURE 6.3A: Equinus foot 45°   **FIGURE 6.3B:** Medial arch 30° (normal)

Equinus deformity is mostly seen in patients of clubfoot, cerebral palsy, polio and sometimes posttraumatic. If there is a shortening of the leg up to 5 cm usually the compensatory equinus should be 45° (Figures 6.3A and B). Equinus deformity can be further classified into the following sub-groups for better understanding—

1. **Equinus deformity up to 45°**
   a. Mild to moderate
   b. Severe
2. **Equinus deformity up to 45° with shortening up to 5 cm**
3. **Equinus >45° and ≤ 60°, when cavus deformity develops according to the extent of equinus**

   a. Mild to moderate
   b. Severe
4. **Equinus >60° (always associated with cavus deformity)**
   a. Mild to moderate
   b. Severe

Equinus Deformity upto 45°; Mild to Moderate

If the deformity is mild to moderate especially in children and adolescents (particularly in cerebral palsy) one full ring and three hole male-post at tibia and one half ring at the base of metatarsal heads are used (Figures 6.4A to C).

One full ring is placed at proximal tibia with two K-wires; the ring is supported by three-hole male-post, which is fixed with one drop wire (Figure 6.4B). Another half ring is placed at forefoot with two K-wires. The forefoot and tibial rings are connected with two telescopic rods. TendoAchilles sub-total tenotomy is done for releasing the tight heel cord after dismantling the forefoot and tibial rings.

The lengthening of tendoAchilles is started @ 1 mm per day from the 7th postoperative day (@ 0.25 mm at 7 am, 11 am, 3 pm and 7 pm). The day of tenotomy should be considered as day 1. Correction of deformity begins by tightening of two telescopic rods. The rate of correction will be mathematically calculated according to Table 7.1.

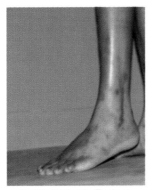

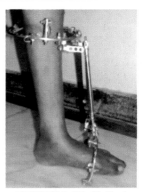

FIGURE 6.4A: Patient before treatment

FIGURE 6.4B: Patient wearing the apparatus

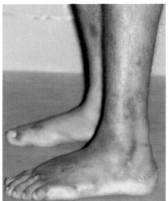

FIGURE 6.4C: Patient after treatment

Sites of Placement of Wires and Rings

Figures 6.5 to 6.7 show the site of placement of wires and rings.

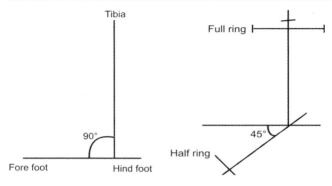

FIGURE 6.5A: Normal foot 90°

FIGURE 6.5B: Sites of placement of rings

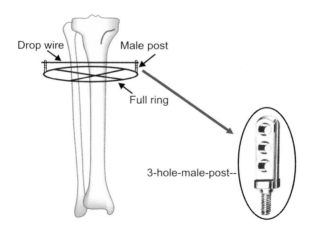

FIGURE 6.6A: One ring with drop wire in tibia

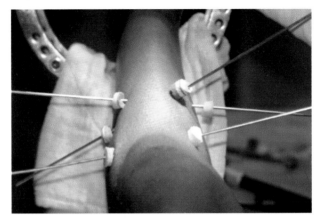

FIGURE 6.6B: Position of K-wires in proximal tibia

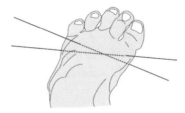

FIGURE 6.6C: Position of K-wires in forefoot

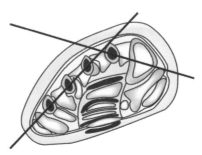

FIGURE 6.6D: Position of K-wires in forefoot
(Transverse section)

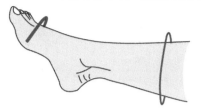

FIGURE 6.6E: Position of rings

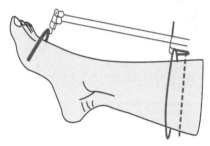

FIGURE 6.6F: Complete frame assembly: two anterior telescopic rods are connecting tibial and forefoot rings

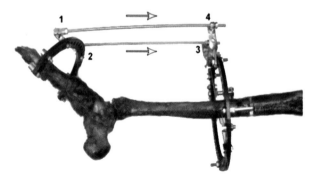

FIGURE 6.7A: Placement of frame on a bone model. Frame assembly on 45° equinus foot. One full ring in tibia and half ring in forefoot connected with two telescopic rods and four hinges (1,2,3,4); two wires in tibial ring, one drop wire connected with tibial ring by three hole male-post, two wires in metatarsals between head and neck

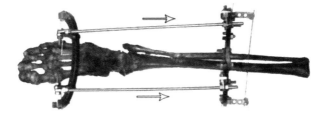

FIGURE 6.7B: Anterior view

Step by Step Procedure for Correcting Mild to Moderate Equinus Foot upto 45° (Figures 6.8A to L)

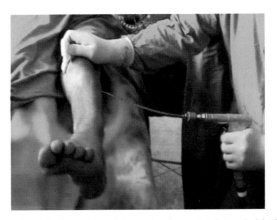

FIGURE 6.8A: Insertion of first wire from the lateral side in left tibia. The first K-wire (1.8 mm) is inserted above the junction of upper and middle third of tibia at about one fingerbreadth lateral and behind the shin of tibia with an inclination of the wire aiming to emerge at the same level just anterior to the medial border. The wire should be parallel to the knee joint.

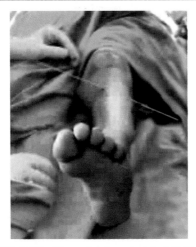

FIGURE 6.8B: First wire inserted in left tibia

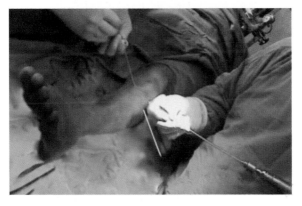

FIGURE 6.8C: Insertion of second wire in left tibia. Second wire is inserted about one fingerbreadth anterior to the palpable anterior border of fibula at a point about 5 mm (thickness of ring 4 mm) below the level of first wire and with an inclination anteriorly aiming the wire to emerge about one fingerbreadth posteromedial to shin of tibia at about the same level

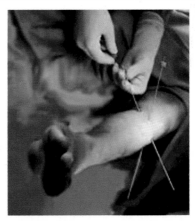

FIGURE 6.8D: Inserted second wire in left tibia

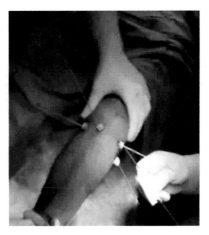

FIGURE 6.8E: Insertion of drop wire in left tibia. A drop wire is being inserted two fingerbreadth above the first proximal wires and two fingerbreadth lateral and behind the shin of tibia aiming the wire to emerge at the same level anterior to the medial border. The wire is horizontal in position

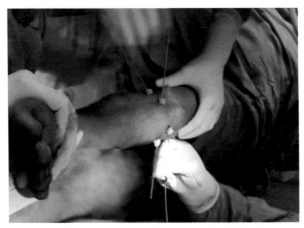

FIGURE 6.8F: Drop wire coming out on the medial side

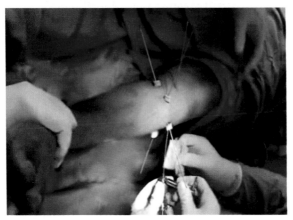

FIGURE 6.8G: Inserted drop wire in left tibia

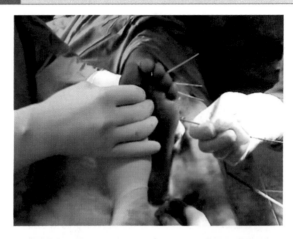

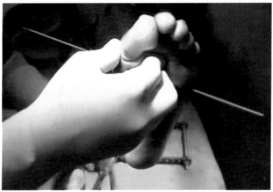

FIGURES 6.8H and I: Insertion of first wire at the base of metatarsal head. The first wire is inserted from the outer side through the distal part of the fifth metatarsal between head and neck and advanced obliquely piercing the fourth and third metatarsal just proximal to their heads to so as to emerge on the surface on the dorsum of the foot

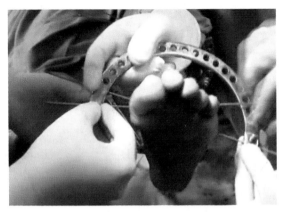

FIGURE 6.8J: The second wire is inserted from dorsal surface base of the third metatarsal with an aim to pierce the central region of the third metatarsal, second metatarsal and first metatarsal. A half forefoot ring is placed below the level of head of metatarsals. The ring is connected to both the wires. The ring should be perpendicular to the forefoot. Tenotomy of tendoAchilles by single stab is performed foot is further plantar flexed 5°

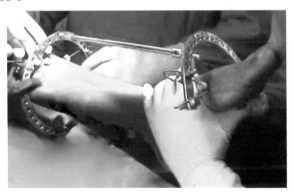

FIGURE 6.8K: Half ring and tibial ring is connected with each other by two telescopic rods and four hinges, both the rods are horizontal and parallel to each other

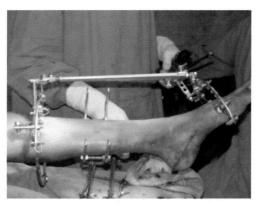

FIGURE 6.8L: Complete frame assembly

Equinus Deformity upto 45°; Severe

Two full rings are placed at tibia (one at the junction of proximal and middle third and another at the junction of middle and distal third) each with two K-wires; half ring is placed on the calcaneus and half ring on the forefoot each with two K-wires. All the rings are connected with each other. Percutaneous subtotal tenotomy of tendoAchilles is done for correction of equinus.

Postoperatively, from 7th day (day 1 is the day of surgery) correction of deformity begins by tightening of two telescopic rods. The rate of correction will be mathematically calculated according to Table 7.1.

Site of Placement of Wire and Rings

Figures 6.9 to 6.19 show the site of placement of wires and rings.

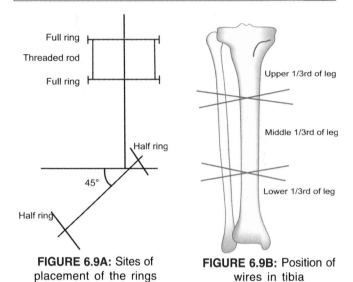

FIGURE 6.9A: Sites of placement of the rings

FIGURE 6.9B: Position of wires in tibia

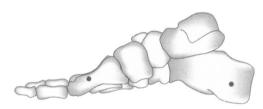

FIGURE 6.9C: Location of wires in the foot, shown by '●'

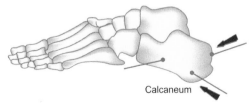

FIGURE 6.9D: Line diagram showing the entry of the first wire and entry and exit of the second wire

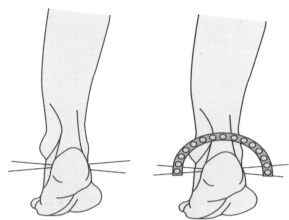

FIGURE 6.9E: The equinus foot viewed from behind showing the passing of two wire in calcaneus

FIGURE 6.9F: The equinus foot from behind with half ring mounted on two K-wire on each side

FIGURES 6.9A to F: Placement of wires and rings

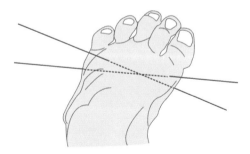

FIGURE 6.10: Position of K-wires in forefoot

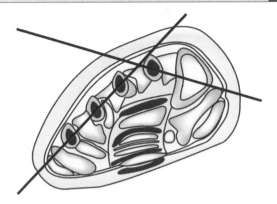

FIGURE 6.11: Transverse section of the forefoot showing the position of K-wires. Note that the first wire passes through the fifth, fourth and third metatarsals while the second one passes through first and second metatarsals

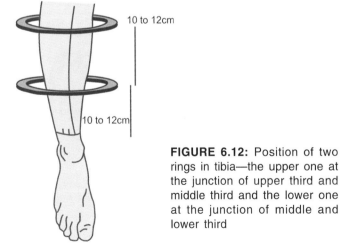

10 to 12cm

10 to 12cm

FIGURE 6.12: Position of two rings in tibia—the upper one at the junction of upper third and middle third and the lower one at the junction of middle and lower third

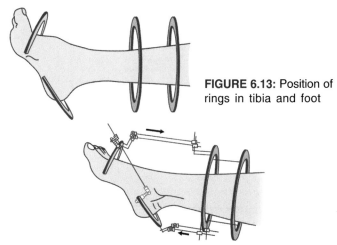

FIGURE 6.13: Position of rings in tibia and foot

FIGURE 6.14: Complete frame assembly. (Two anterior threaded rods connecting the tibial and forefoot rings and two posterior threaded rods, connecting the tibial and calcaneal rings), complete frame assembly shown in models to clarify the positions of wires, rings and connecting rods

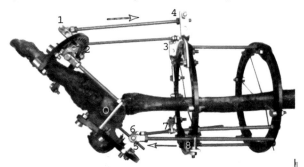

FIGURE 6.15: Placement of frame in a bone model with equinus deformity 45°. Two full rings in tibia, one half ring in forefoot and one half ring in calcaneus. Tibial and forefoot rings have been connected with two threaded rods and four hinges (1,2,3,4). Tibial and calcaneal rings have been connected with two threaded rods and four hinges (5,6,7,8)

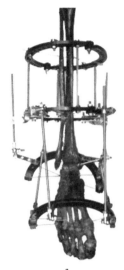

FIGURE 6.16: Anterior view of configuration

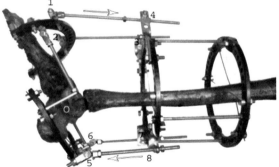

FIGURE 6.17: The 45° of equinus (Figure 6.15) 15° has been corrected leaving behind 30° equinus as residual. By loosing the posterior rods and tightening the anterior rods the equinus has been corrected by 15 degrees. In the process of correction of equinus the forefoot ring moves along a circular path, the center of which lies at the axis of the ankle joint. Correspondingly the short lever arm of the foot, i.e. the calcaneus moves downwards

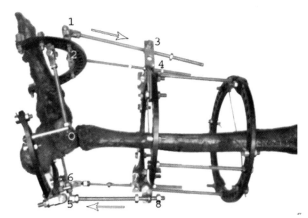

FIGURE 6.18: The 45° of equinus (Figure 6.23A) 30° has been corrected leaving behind 15° equinus as residual

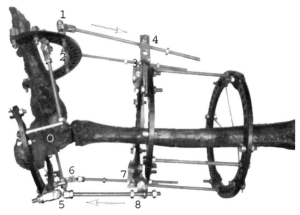

FIGURE 6.19: Equinus fully corrected. During correction of equinus foot the forefoot ring goes upward along the circular path, the anterior threaded rods goes posterior (downward) whose motion is controlled by the loose hinges (1,2,3,4) and the posterior threaded rods also goes posterior (downward) whose motion is controlled by the loose hinges (5,6,7,8)

Step by Step Procedure for Equinus 45°
(Figures 6.20A to Y)

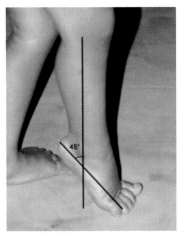

FIGURE 6.20A: Preoperative

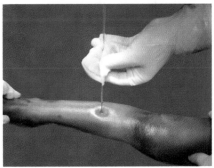

FIGURE 6.20B: Insertion of first wire from the lateral side in right tibia. The first K-wire (1.8 mm) is inserted at the junction of upper and middle third of tibia at about one fingerbreadth lateral and behind the shin of tibia with an inclination of the wire aiming to emerge at the same level just anterior to the medial border. The wire should be parallel to the knee joint

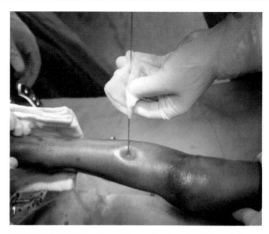

FIGURE 6.20C: Insertion of wire in right tibia

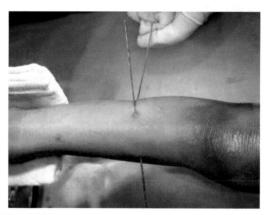

FIGURE 6.20D: Insertion of second wire in right tibia. Second wire is inserted about one fingerbreadth anterior to the palpable anterior border of fibula at a point about 5 mm (thickness of ring 4 mm) below the level of the first wire and with an inclination anteriorly aiming the wire to emerge about one fingerbreadth posteromedial to shin of tibia at about the same level

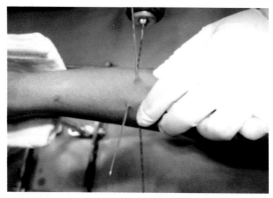

FIGURE 6.20E: Insertion of second wire in tibia

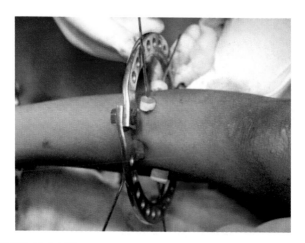

FIGURE 6.20F: Ring fixation in tibia. A full ring of optimal diameter is connected to both the wires by wire fixation bolts, one wire should be on one side of the ring and the second should be on the other side. The anterior junction of the ring should be at the shin of tibia

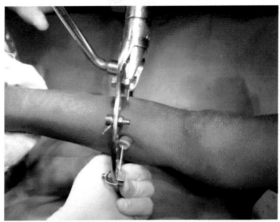

FIGURE 6.20G: Tensioning of wires in tibia. Each wire is tensioned from anteromedial and antero-lateral ends of the wire; while the posteromedial and posterolateral ends are kept fixed. First wire is tensioned from anterolateral side while the postero-medial end of the wire is fixed

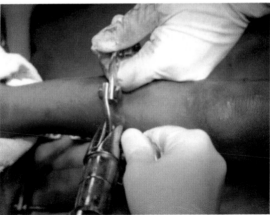

FIGURE 6.20H: Tensioning of wires in tibia. The second wire is tensioned from anteromedial side while posterolateral end of the wire is fixed

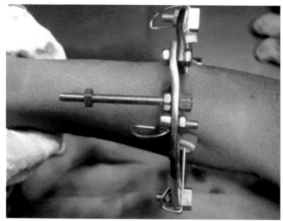

FIGURE 6.20I: Ring with threaded rod in tibia. The first threaded rod should be fixed in the first hole medial to the anterior junction. The length of the rod should be such so that the second full ring could be placed about 10-12 cm above the ankle joint, i.e. at the junction of lower third and middle third

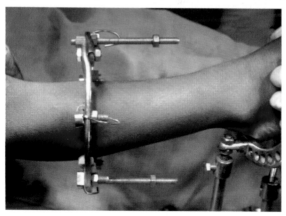

FIGURE 6.20J: Ring with threaded rods in right tibia. The second threaded rod should be fixed in the first hole lateral to the posterior junction

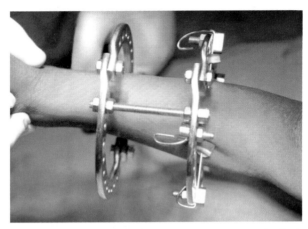

FIGURE 6.20K: The second ring is connected to both the threaded rods

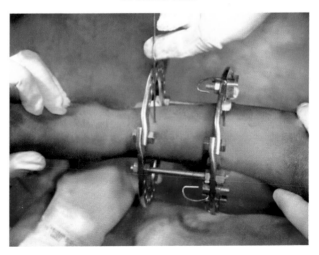

FIGURE 6.20L: Insertion of first wire for second ring of tibia

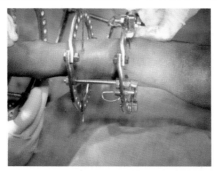

FIGURE 6.20M: The first wire of this set is inserted through fibula and passed through the tibia with an inclination aiming the wire to emerge one fingerbreadth anteromedial to the shin of tibia

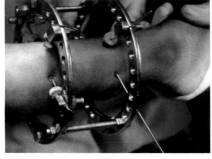

FIGURE 6.20N: Insertion of second wire for second ring of tibia. The point of selection for inserting the second wire should be ascertained cautiously. The space between the anterior border of tibia and fibula is divided into three equal zones. The anterior zone contains neurovascular structures and tendons. The middle zone is more or less safer containing mostly the muscular part. At about 5 mm (thickness of ring 4 mm) below the level of the first wire, the second wire is inserted through the safe corridor of middle zone into the tibia with an inclination to emerge just anterior to the medial border of tibia. The wires are fixed and tensioned as done in the proximal ring. Both rings are always fixed with four threaded rods

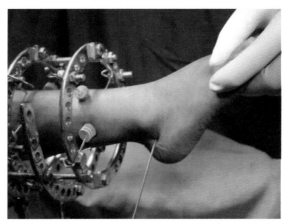

FIGURE 6.20O: Insertion of first wire in calcaneus. The first wire is inserted on the outer surface of calcaneum about 1 cm above its inferior surface and 1 cm distal to the attachment of tendoAchilles. The wire is advanced with an inclination anteromedially aiming to emerge on the medial surface of the calcaneum two fingers breadth below the medial malleolus (to avoid any damage to neurovascular bundle)

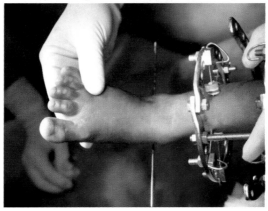

FIGURE 6.20P: Inserted wire in calcaneus

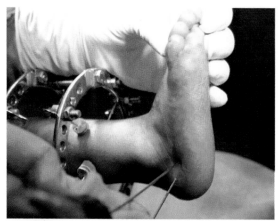

FIGURE 6.20Q: The second wire is inserted one fingerbreadth distal to the entry point of the first wire and is advanced obliquely posteromedially to emerge about one fingerbreadth behind the first wire in the same level

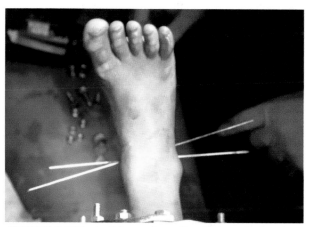

FIGURE 6.20R: In this configuration the *angle forming* between the two wires is more or less 30°

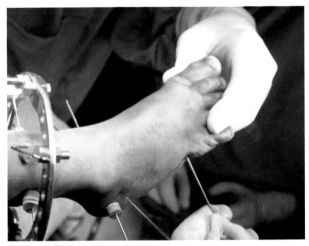

FIGURE 6.20S: Insertion of first wire in the base of metatarsal head first wire is inserted from the lateral side through the distal part of the 5th metatarsal between head and neck and advanced obliquely piercing the fourth and third metatarsal just proximal to their head to emerge on the surface on the dorsum of the foot

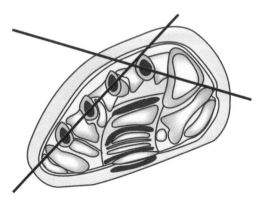

FIGURE 6.20T: Position of K-wires through the base of metatarsal head

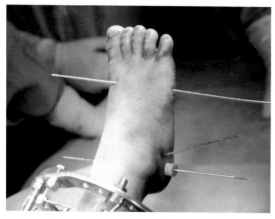

FIGURE 6.20U: Inserted first wire in metatarsal head

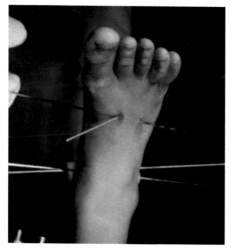

FIGURE 6.20V: Inserted wires in forefoot. The second wire is inserted on the distal region of medial surface of the first metatarsal just proximal to its head and advances obliquely to pierce through the second metatarsal and ultimately emerges on the dorsum of foot

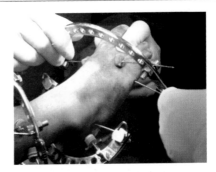

FIGURE 6.20W: Placement of half ring in forefoot. Half calcaneal ring is placed at the calcaneum, the ring should be parallel to the heel. In case of varus or valgus deformity, the orientation of ring should be according to the deformity. A half forefoot ring is placed below the level of head of metatarsals, the ring should be perpendicular to the forefoot. The calcaneal and forefoot rings are connected to each other with two threaded rods

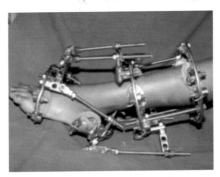

FIGURE 6.20X: Complete frame assembly. Foot assembly is connected with the distal tibial ring. The forefoot half ring is connected anteriorly to the distal tibial ring with two threaded rods and four hinges and the calcaneal half ring is connected with the distal tibial ring posteriorly with two threaded rods and four hinges. All the four rods should be horizontal and parallel to each other

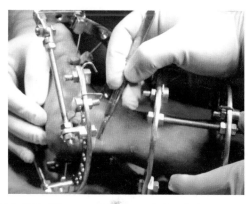

FIGURE 6.20Y: All connecting threaded rods between foot and tibia are dismantled and percutaneous subtotal tendoAchilles tenotomy is performed. The frame is reassembled with 2 mm overriding of the tendoAchilles cut ends by increasing the equinus

Equinus Deformity up to 45° with Shortened Limb up to 5 cm

In the first step, the **fibular osteotomy** is done above the junction of middle third and lower third of the leg keeping enough space away from the site of passing the K-wire at the junction of middle and lower third and also there should be enough space from the ring to avoid the superimposition of the metallic shadow of the ring on the underlined regenerating fibula, which otherwise will interfere with proper monitoring of the fibular regeneration during the lengthening procedure (see Figure 6.21B). In poliomyelitis the regeneration is on the whole poor, hence it is better to perform the fibular osteotomy in mid shaft region.

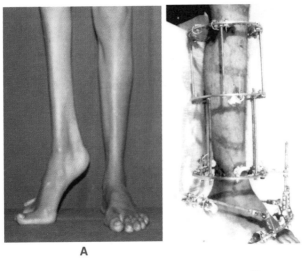

A

B

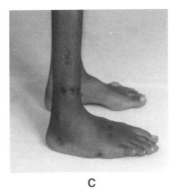

C

FIGURE 6.21A to C: A. Patient before treatment; B. Patient wearing the apparatus; C. Patient after treatment

For performing fibular osteotomy 1-2 cm of longitudinal incision is given over the fibula at the selected site. A 10 to 15 mm osteotome is inserted in longitudinal direction to over the fibula, and then osteotome is rotated by 90° with 10 to 15° of obliquity. Fixing the osteotome firmly it is hammered over to cut the fibula obliquely (Figures 6.22A toC)

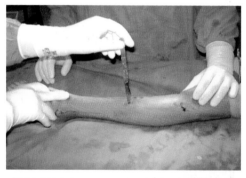

A

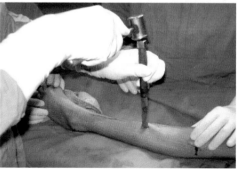

B

FIGURES 6.22A AND B

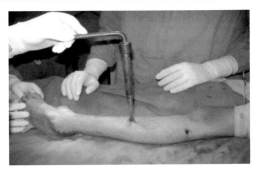

C

FIGURES 6.22A to C: A. Insertion of BP Blade; B. Insertion of osteotome; C. Rotation of osteotome 90°

In the second step, frame construction is done by placing three rings in tibia. Proximal ring is fixed with two K-wires, one from head of fibula another from anterolateral surface of tibia. The middle ring is fixed with two K-wires passed at about the junction of upper and middle third of tibia. The remaining distal ring is fixed with two K-wires passed at about the junction of middle and lower third of tibia. All the rings are connected to each other by four connecting rods. The half calcaneal ring is connected with two K-wires passed through calcaneus. This calcaneal ring is connected to the distal tibial ring by two hinges and connecting rods. The half forefoot ring is secured with two K-wires which have been already passed. Then the calcaneal and forefoot half rings are connected each other by two hinges and threaded rods. The forefoot ring is also connected to the distal tibial full ring by two threaded rods and four hinges.

In the third step, the connecting threaded rods of proximal and middle tibial rings are dismantled to facilitate the **corticotomy of tibia** in the upper region just distal to the tibial tuberosity. After the corticotomy the disconnected rods are reconnected. It is wise to confirm the completion of corticotomy under image intensifier by visualizing the gap created of about 2 to 3 mm at the corticotomy site by distracting the four connecting rods between the proximal and middle ring (Figure 6.23).

For performing corticotomy of tibia 1.5 cm longitudinal incision is given at one fingerbreadth below and lateral to the tibial tuberosity. The incision is deepened by stabing the BP blade up to the bone. Then a 5 to 10 mm size

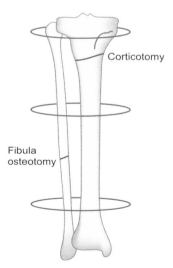

FIGURE 6.23: Position of rings, corticotomy

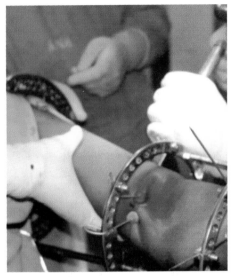

FIGURE 6.24: Photograph of placement of osteotome

osteotome is inserted longitudinally up to the bone (Figure 6.24). After firmly feeling the bone the osteotome is rotated by 90°. First the anteromedial cortex of tibia is cut then osteotome is slightly withdrawn and anterolateral cortex of tibia is cut. While cutting the tibial cortex 1/3rd of the edge of the osteotome always remain out side the bone and should be felt by finger tip to monitor the cutting of the cortex. The posterior cortex is broken by performing rotational movements by holding the proximal and middle rings. However, the internal rotational movement of the proximal ring should not be done to avoid the damage to the lateral popliteal nerve. All does not accept the original concept of avoiding interference with the medullary cavity by the osteotome. Considering this concept only the corticotomy is being performed even by the Giggly saw in one stage through and through (Paley 2002).

In the fourth step the threaded connecting rods between distal tibial, calcaneal and forefoot rings are dismantled to facilitate **percutaneous tendoAchilles lengthening** either by single stab or two-stab incision according to indication, expertise and experience (in spastic single stab incision and gradual lengthening should be preferred). After completion of lengthening the dismantled rods are reconnected.

Postoperatively, on 7th day lengthening of tibia and correction of equinus are performed simultaneously.

Site of Placements of Wires and Rings

Figures 6.25 to 6.31 show the site of placement of wires and rings:

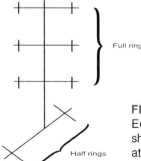

Full rings

Half rings

FIGURE 6.25: Ring placement in Equinus deformity up to 45° with shortening up to 5 cm, three full rings at tibia, one half ring at forefoot and one half ring in calcaneus

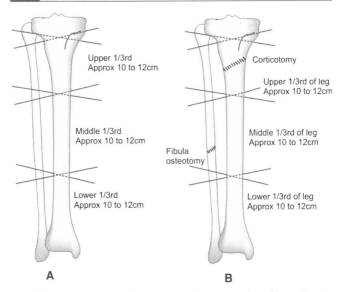

FIGURES 6.26A and B: A. Wire placement in tibia and site of corticotomy

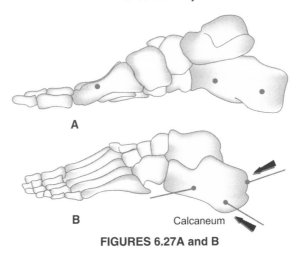

FIGURES 6.27A and B

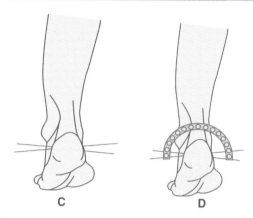

FIGURES 6.27A to D: A. Sites of wire location in calcaneum and first metatarsal viewed from medial side; B. Direction of wires through calcaneum from lateral side; C. Wire passed through calcaneum viewed from posterior side; D. Wires (as in C2.7C) fixed on half ring

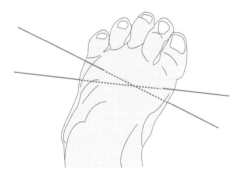

FIGURE 6.28A: Position of K- wires in forefoot

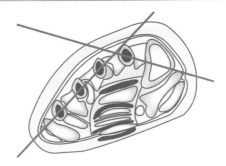

FIGURE 6.28B: Position of K- wires in forefoot (transverse section)

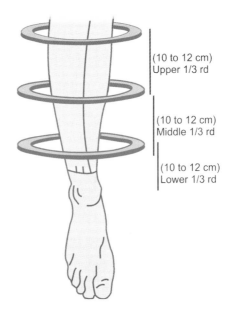

(10 to 12 cm)
Upper 1/3 rd

(10 to 12 cm)
Middle 1/3 rd

(10 to 12 cm)
Lower 1/3 rd

FIGURE 6.29: Position of three rings in tibia

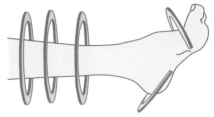

FIGURE 6.30: Position of rings in tibia and foot

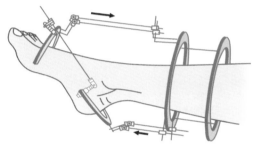

FIGURE 6.31: Complete frame assembly

Step by Step Procedure for Equinus with Shortening 3 cm: Figures 6.32A to AQ)

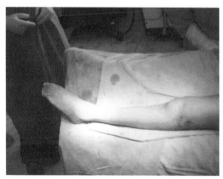

FIGURE 6.32A: Equinus with 3cm shortening

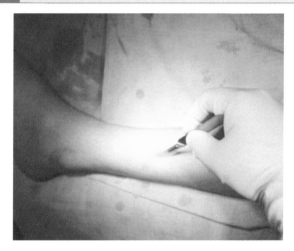

FIGURE 6.32B: Osteotomy of fibula above the junction of middle-third and lower-third of fibula

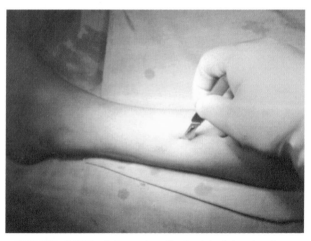

FIGURE 6.32C: 1-2 cm longitudinal incision is given anteriorily over fibula

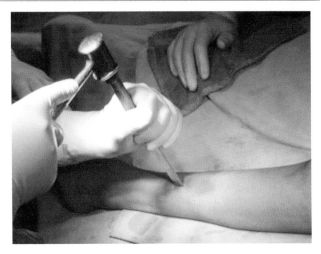

FIGURE 6.32D: 10 mm osteotome inserted in longitudinal direction over fibula

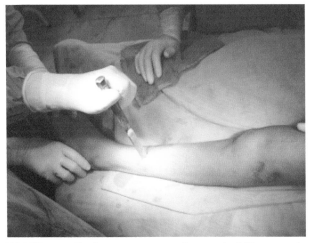

FIGURE 6.32E: Osteotome rotated towards 90° to cut the bone in 10°-15° oblique direction

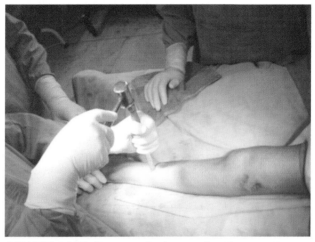

FIGURE 6.32F: Bone cut by hammering the osteotome

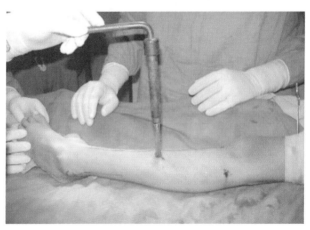

FIGURE 6.32G: Rotation of osteotome to disengage the fragment

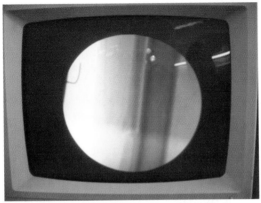

FIGURE 6.32H: One may confirm fibular osteotomy under image

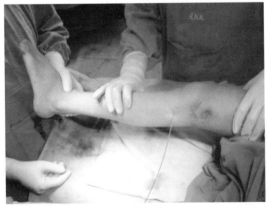

FIGURE 6.32I: After fibular osteotomy reference wire should be passed first from the anterolateral region of the flare of lateral condyle of tibia (one fingerbreadth in front and one finger-breadth above the head of fibula — approx 14 mm below the joint line) to emerge on the same level through the flare of medial condyle of tibia. The wire should be tilted proximally 5° on the medial side to compensate the valgus which may develop during lengthening

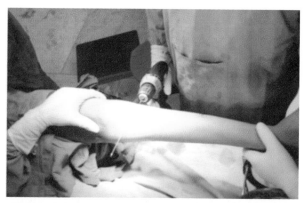

FIGURE 6.32J: The wire should emerge 5° proximal on medial side

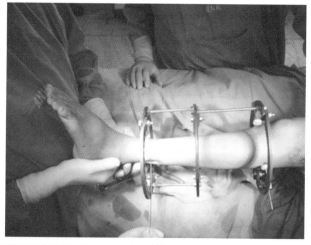

FIGURE 6.32K: Preassembled Ilizarov frame is placed over the limb with the patient supine. The frame is fixed to the proximal reference wire. The second reference 1.8 mm wire is inserted through lower third of fibula and passed through tibia with an inclination aiming the wire to emerge one fingerbreadth posteromedial to the shin of tibia. The frame is attached to the second reference wire

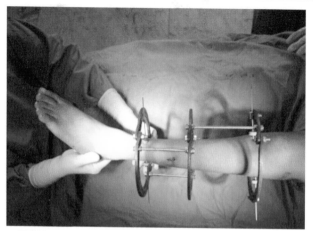

FIGURE 6.32L: Distal tibial wires emerging on the anteromedial surface

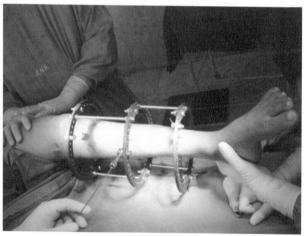

FIGURE 6.32M: 6.5 mm Schanz screw is inserted on the medial surface anterior to the medial border. The guide wire is passed through drill sleeve

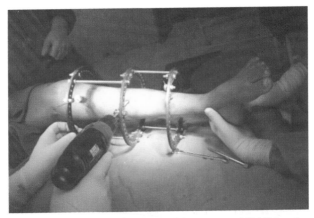

FIGURE 6.32N: Drilling is done by 3.5 mm drill-bit to place the Schanz screw

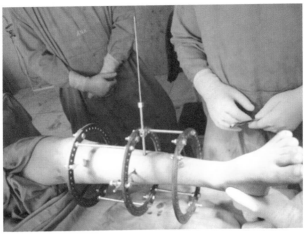

FIGURE 6.32O: 5 mm Schanz screw is inserted; another Schanz screw is placed on the medial surface closed to the shin of tibia over the guide wire

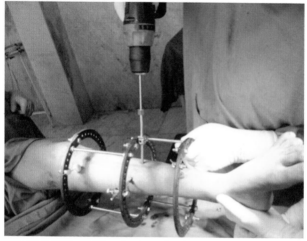

FIGURE 6.32P: Drilling is done by 3.5 mm drill-bit to insert the Schanz screw at the shin of tibia

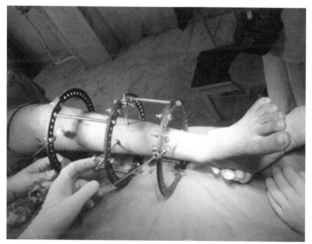

FIGURE 6.32Q: 5 mm Schanz screw is inserted. Note: *Instead of two Schanz screws, one Schanz screw and one wire can be passed*

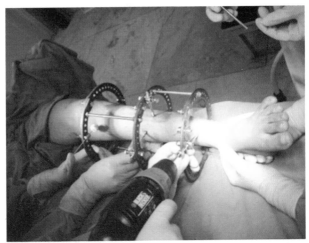

FIGURE 6.32R: Drilling is done by 3.5 mm drill bit to insert the Schanz screw on the medial surface of tibia, anterior to the medial border

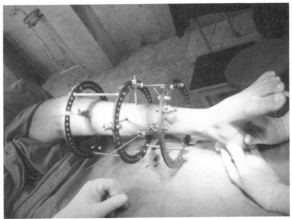

FIGURE 6.32S: First, a guide wire is passed to locate the point for inserting the second Schanz screw on the medial surface of the tibia proximal to the ring with the help of two hole block for half pin

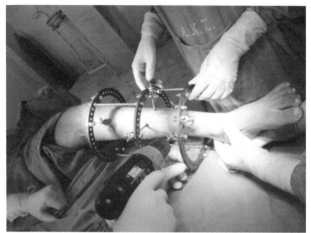

FIGURE 6.32T: Drilling is done by 3.5 mm drill bit to insert the Schanz screw Note: *Instead of one wire and two Schanz screws, two or three wires can be passed*

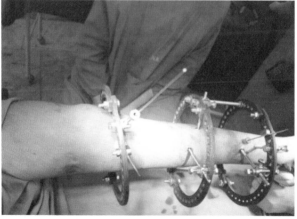

FIGURE 6.32U: Ring is tilted 5° anticlockwise to compensate procurvatum which may develop during lengthening. Second K wire passes from the head of fibula and comes out from anteromedial side

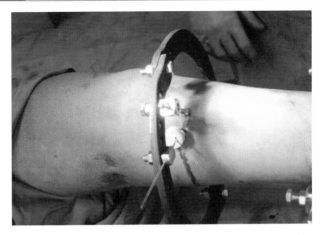

FIGURE 6.32V: Schanz screw is inserted at the same place after drilling with cannulated drill bit up to the head of fibula

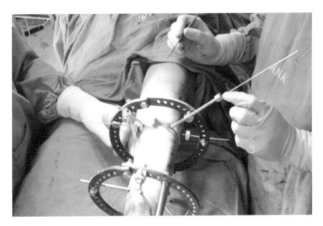

FIGURE 6.32W: Guide wire for the Schanz screw on anterolateral surface

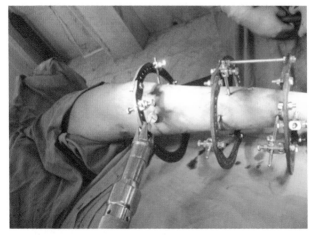

FIGURE 6.32X: Schanz screw insertion and tensioning of wire

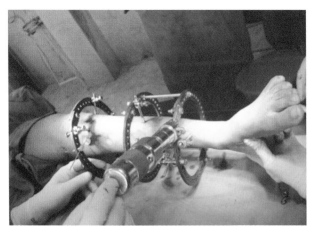

FIGURE 6.32Y: Tensioning of distal K-wire

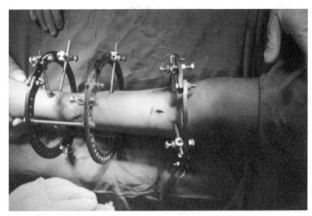

FIGURE 6.32Z: 10 to 15 mm longitudinal incision is given 1 cm below and lateral to tibial tuberosity

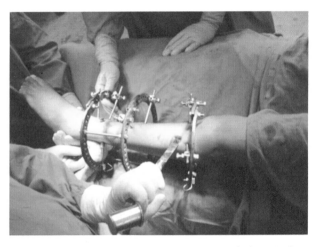

FIGURE 6.32AA: 5-10 mm osteotome is inserted longitudinally from lateral side up to the bone

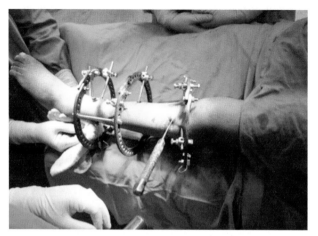

FIGURE 6.32AB: Osteotome is rotated 90°

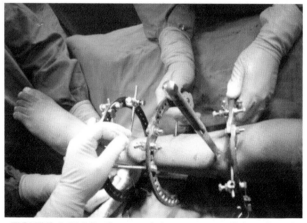

FIGURE 6.32AC: Cortex of the anteromedial surface is osteotomized

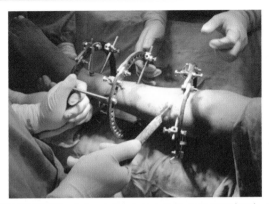

FIGURE 6.32AD: Anterolateral cortex is osteotomized, cortical edge is cut in the anteromedial and posterolateral region of bone to avoid damage to bone marrow, with the help of wrench. The unosteotomized part of cortical layer is broken by rotating the osteotome in different directions. In some cases, additional proximal and middle rings are rotated opposite to each other. Care should be taken not to rotate proximal ring in medial direction, because of stretch the peroneal nerve. Two bone ends are then separated and distracted 2-3 mm apart to confirm the complete corticotomy

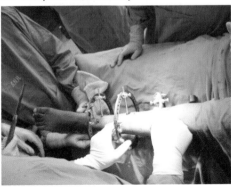

FIGURE 6.32AE: Rotation of proximal ring in anti-clock wise and medial ring clock wise for breaking the bone and to avoid stretching of nerve

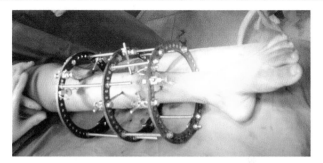

FIGURE 6.32AF: Frame assembly of tibia

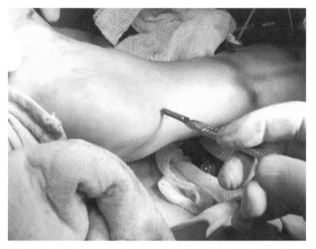

FIGURE 6.32AG: Lengthening of tendoAchilles is performed (one fingerbreadth above the insertion of tendoAchilles a no. 15 BP blade is introduced in the center of the tendoAchilles parallel to its fibers)

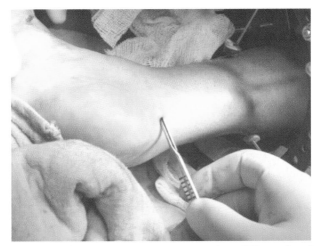

FIGURE 6.32AH: The BP blade is turned medially cutting the medial half of the Achilles tendon, and the scalpel is withdrawn

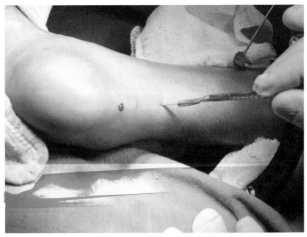

FIGURE 6.32AI: The BP blade is again inserted in the center of the Achilles tendon two fingerbreadth above the first step

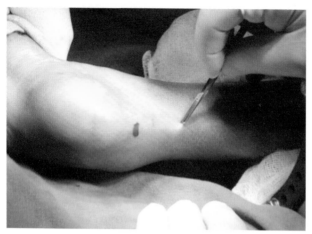

FIGURE 6.32AJ: BP blade is turn 90° laterally cutting the lateral half of the Achilles tendon

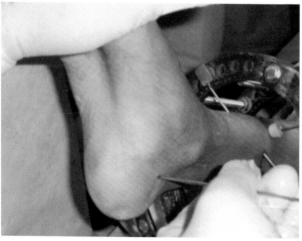

FIGURE 6.32AK: Posterior tibial artery pulsation is felt, posterior tibial nerve is palpated. On the medial surface of calcaneous, the first 1.8 mm K-wire is inserted one fingerbreadth above the under surface of calcaneous and one fingerbreadth in front of tendoAchilles

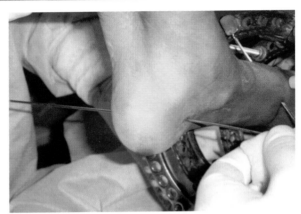

FIGURE 6.32AL: The wire is advanced with an inclination anterolaterally at an inclination of 30° aiming to emerge on the lateral surface of calcaneus one and half fingerbreadth below the lateral malleolus

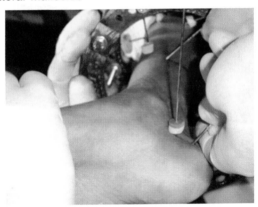

FIGURE 6.32AM: Second wire is inserted 1cm anterior to the first wire and 1cm above the inferior surface of calcaneus the wire is advanced laterally to emerge 1cm above the inferior surface and 1cm distal to attachment of tendoAchilles (the second wire is inserted with cautious not to damage any neurovascular bundle)

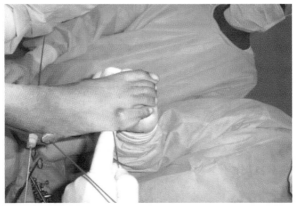

FIGURE 6.32AN: First 1.5 mm K-wire is inserted from the outer side through the distal part of the fifth metatarsal between head and neck

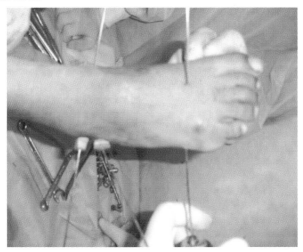

FIGURE 6.32AO: The wire is advanced obliquely piercing the fifth, fourth and third metatarsal just proximal to their heads to emerge on the surface on the dorsum of the foot

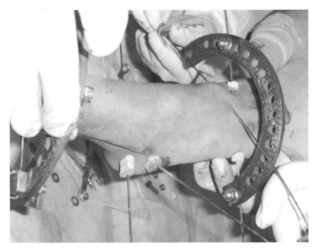

FIGURE 6.32AP: The second wire is inserted on the medial surface in the distal first metatarsal just proximal to its head and advances obliquely to emerge on the dorsum of foot after piercing through second metatarsal. A half ring is attached to the K-wires, the ring should be perpendicular to the forefoot

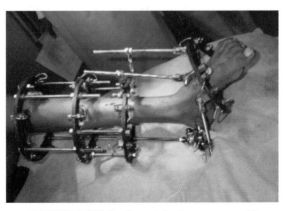

FIGURE 6.32AQ: Complete frame assembly

Equinus (Equinocavus) Deformity >45° and ≤ 60°; Mild to Moderate

If the equinus deformity is more than 45° it is usually associated with cavus deformity of foot. Two full rings are placed at tibia with two K-wires, a half ring is placed at calcaneus with two K-wires and a half ring is placed at forefoot with two K-wires, tendoAchilles tenotomy is done for equinus correction (Figures 6.33 to 6.35).

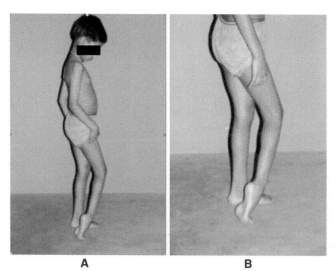

A   **B**

FIGURES 6.33A and B: 5 year old cerebral palsy child with 60° equinus

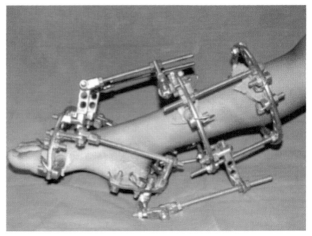

FIGURE 6.34: Postoperative frame assembly

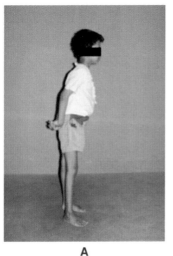

A

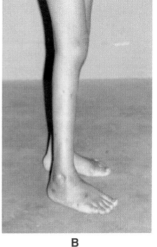

B

FIGURES 6.35A and B: Full correction achieved

Site of Placements of Wires and Rings

Figures 6.36 to 6.43 show the site of placement of wires and rings:

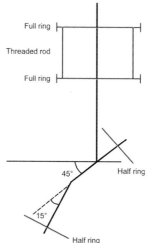

FIGURE 6.36: Mild to moderate equinocavus 45° equinus + 15° cavus. Ring placement in equinocavus deformity > 45° and ≤60°

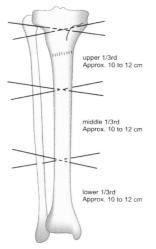

FIGURE 6.37: Position of wires in tibia

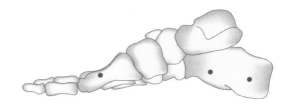

FIGURE 6.38: Wire location in foot

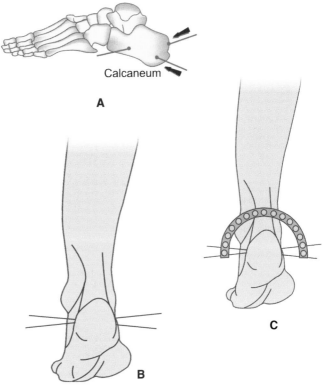

Calcaneum

A

B

C

FIGURES 6.39A to C: Wires in calcaneus

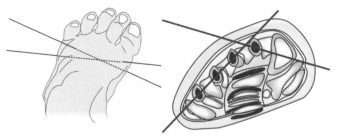

FIGURES 6.40A and B: A. Position of K-wires in forefoot; B. Position of K-wires in forefoot (Transverse section)

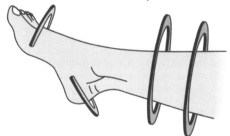

FIGURE 6.41: Position of rings

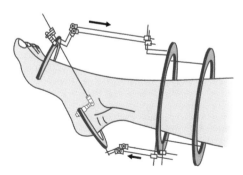

FIGURE 6.42: Complete frame assembly

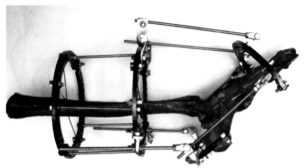

FIGURE 6.43A: Frame assembly on a bone model of equinocavus deformity 60°. Two full rings in tibia, one half ring in forefoot and one half ring in calcaneus. Tibial and forefoot rings connected with two anterior threaded rods and four hinges. Tibial and calcaneal rings connected with two posterior threaded rods and four hinges

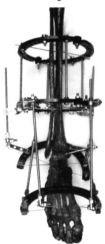

FIGURE 6.43B: Top view, two anterior threaded rods are parallel to each other and two posterior rods are also parallel to each other

Equinus (Equinocavus) Deformitty >45° and ≤ 60°; Severe

For correction of severe equinocavus two full rings at tibia, one half ring at calcaneus, one half ring at apex of cavus and one full ring at forefoot is required.

First, we correct 45° equinus deformity. The rest of the cavus deformity is corrected by distraction between ring of midfoot and forefoot and hindfoot and forefoot (Figures 6.44 to 6.47).

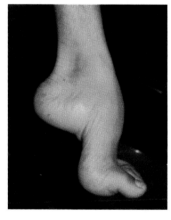

FIGURE 6.44: Preoperative

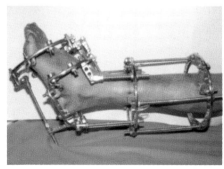

FIGURE 6.45: Postoperative frame assembly

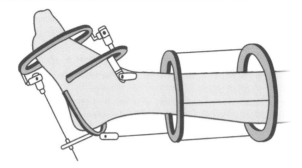

FIGURE 6.46: Postoperative schematic diagram

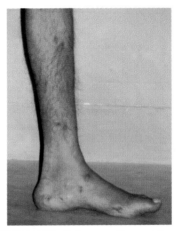

FIGURE 6.47: Full correction achieved

Frame Construction

Two full rings in tibia each with two 1.8 mm K-wires, one half ring in calcaneus with two 1.5 mm K-wires, one half ring in midfoot with two 1.5 mm K-wires, and one full ring in forefoot with two 1.5 mm K-wires are required (wires in foot ring should not be tensioned).

Both tibial rings are connected with each other with four threaded rods, tibial and calcaneal rings are connected with two threaded rods and four hinges, calcaneal and forefoot rings are connected with two threaded rods and posts, midfoot and forefoot rings are connected with two threaded rods and posts, and forefoot and tibial rings are connected with two threaded rods and four hinges.

Anterior threaded rods connecting forefoot and tibial rings are placed in an angle in upward direction from distal to proximal. The angles of upward direction of threaded rods will depend upon the angle of cavus, in the same way posterior threaded rods are placed in upward direction form distal to proximal (see Figure 6.58).

Threaded rods between foot assembly and tibial assembly are dismantled; tendoAchilles subtotal tenotomy and plantar fasciotomy is performed and threaded rods are reconnected. First, equinus is corrected (correction is started on 7th day by tightening of the anterior threaded rods and loosening of posterior threaded rods) according to the geometrical formula of tendoAchilles lengthening as shown in Table 7.1 gradually the equinus up to 45° is corrected but care must be taken for the joint space of the ankle joint.

Correction of Cavus

Now the assembly configuration is changed. Mid tarsal half ring and calcaneal ring is connected with the tibial ring; distraction is done between calcaneal ring and forefoot ring and mid tarsal ring and forefoot ring. The soft tissue distraction can be done up to 3 mm per day. The distraction on the plantar surface is double than that of the dorsal surface (e.g. if the distraction on the dorsal surface is 1.5 mm than distraction on plantar surface will be 3 mm per day). The distraction is continued until full correction is achieved.

Site of Placements of Wires and Rings

Figures 6.48 to 6.59 show the site of placement of wires and rings:

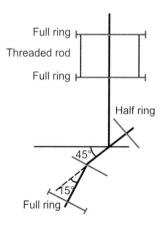

FIGURE 6.48: Ring placement in equinocavus (severe)

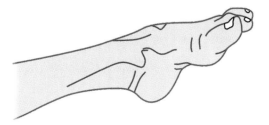

FIGURE 6.49: Sketch of equinocavus foot

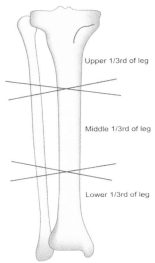

Upper 1/3rd of leg

Middle 1/3rd of leg

Lower 1/3rd of leg

FIGURE 6.50: Position of wires in tibia

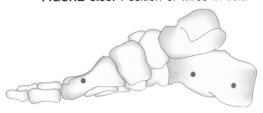

FIGURE 6.51: Wire location in foot

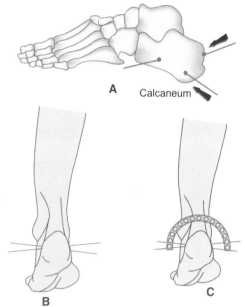

A   Calcaneum

B   C

FIGURES 6.52A to C: Wires in calcaneus

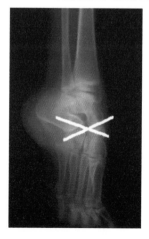

FIGURE 6.53: Pre-operative X-ray
with wire position

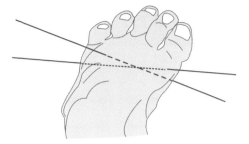

FIGURE 6.54: Position of K- wires in forefoot

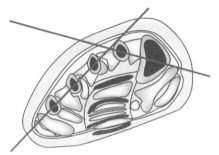

FIGURE 6.55: Position of K-wires in forefoot
(Transverse section)

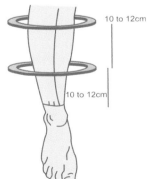

FIGURE 6.56: Position of two
rings in tibia

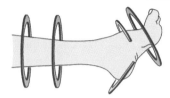

FIGURE 6.57: Position of rings in tibia and foot

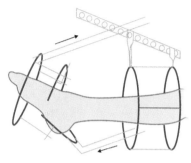

FIGURE 6.58: Frame assembly for correction of equinus, anterior threaded rods connecting the forefoot and tibial ring placed in an angle in upward direction from distal to proximal, similarly posterior threaded rods placed in upward direction from distal to proximal

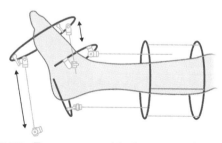

FIGURE 6.59: Frame assembly for correction of cavus. Distraction between calcaneus and forefoot ring, midfoot ring and forefoot ring, distraction on the planter surface is double than that of the dorsal surface

Equinus (Equinocavus) Deformity >60°; Mild to Moderate

The equinus deformity is corrected first followed by the correction of cavus (Figures 6.60 to 6.62). The whole procedure of correction is same as in equinocavus deformity >45 and ≤ 60 degree discussed previously (Figures 6.58 and 6.59).

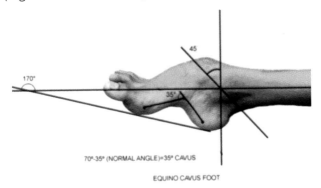

170°

45

35°

70°-35° (NORMAL ANGLE)=35° CAVUS

EQUINO CAVUS FOOT

FIGURE 6.60: 80°Equinocavus foot (Equinus 45°, Cavus 35°)

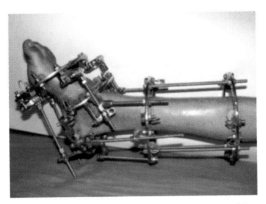

FIGURE 6.61: Postoperative frame assembly

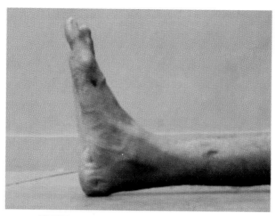

FIGURE 6.62: Full correction achieved

Site of Placements of Wires and Rings

Figures 6.63 to 6.71 show the site of placement of wires and rings:

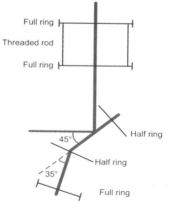

Equinus >60°)
Equinus 45° +Cavus 35°

FIGURE 6.63: Ring placement in equinus >60°

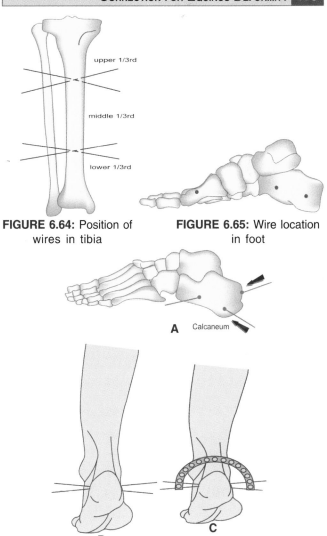

FIGURE 6.64: Position of wires in tibia

FIGURE 6.65: Wire location in foot

FIGURES 6.66A to C: Wires in calcaneus

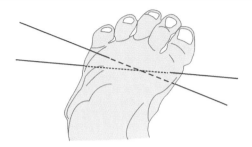

FIGURE 6.67: Position of K-wires in forefoot

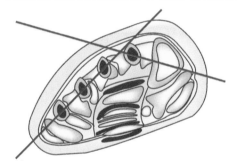

FIGURE 6.68: Position of K-wires in forefoot (transverse section)

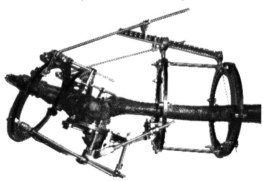

FIGURE 6.69: Placement of frame in a bony model showing equinocavus 65°(45+20)

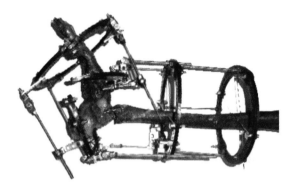

FIGURE 6.70: Equinus 45° corrected and rest of the cavus has to be corrected

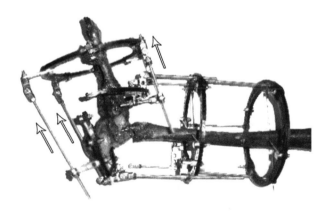

FIGURE 6.71: Cavus is corrected by distraction between rings of mid foot and forefoot, and rings of hind foot and forefoot

Equinocavus >60° Severe (Figures 6.72 and 6.73)

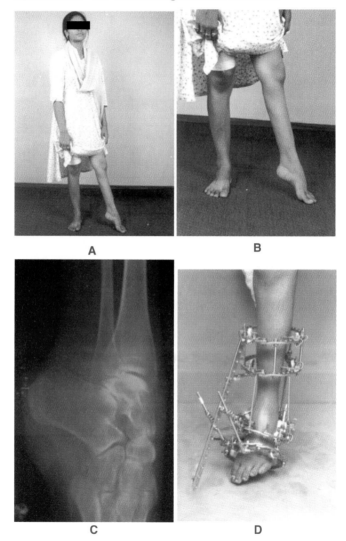

A

B

C

D

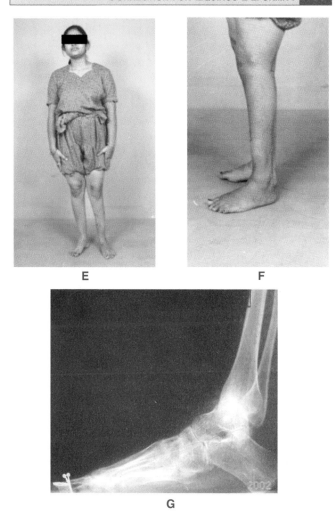

FIGURES 6.72 A to G: A case of pre an post treatment of equinocavus of 45° (severe). A and B Patient before treatment; C. Pre operative X-ray; D. Patient wearing frame; E. Patient after treatment; F and G. Final X-ray after removing frame

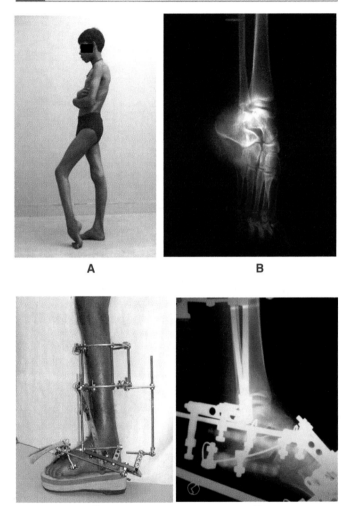

A

B

C

D

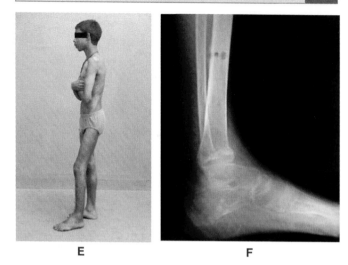

E   F

FIGURES 6.73A to F: A case of pre and post treatment of equinocavus of 60° (severe). A. Patient before treatment; B. Pre operative X-ray; C. Patient wearing frame; D. X-ray with frame; E. Patient after treatment; F. Final X-ray after removing frame

Two full rings are placed at tibia each with 2 K-wires, a half ring is placed at calcaneus with two K-wires, another full ring at apex of mid tarsal region with two K-wires and a full ring are placed at forefoot with two K-wires and tendoAchilles tenotomy is done for correction.

First we correct the 45° equinus deformity. The rest of the cavus deformity is corrected by distraction between the forefoot and midfoot via forefoot ring and midfoot ring. Distraction between midfoot and hindfoot is also given (Figure 6.75).

Site of Placement of Wires and Rings

Figures 6.74 and 6.75 show the site of placement of wires and rings:

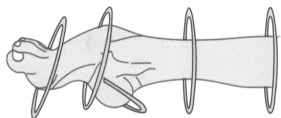

FIGURE 6.74: Position of rings in tibia and foot

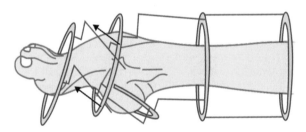

FIGURE 6.75: Complete frame assembly

Chapter 7

Kinematics

KINEMATICS FOR CORRECTION OF THE EQUINUS FOOT

Movements of the whole foot primarily take place at the ankle joint; of course, simultaneous movements also take place at other joints.

Axis of Movements at the Ankle Joint

The axis of the ankle joint in coronal plane is the line joining the tip of the medial malleolus to the tip of the lateral malleolus. It is inclined downward from medial to the lateral side by an average inclination angle of 12°, because the lateral malleolus is downward and posterior to the medial malleolus (Figures 7.1A and B).

Causes of Equinus Deformity

1. Paralytic imbalance of plantar flexor muscles and dorsiflexor muscles, the former being stronger, polio being the commonest cause.
2. In spastics, persistent spasticity of calf muscles mainly the tendoAchilles gradually leading to equinus.
3. Compensatory equinus developing in shortening of the limb
4. Injury and diseases affecting the normal bony architecture of ankle and foot.

With passage of time variable stiffness of the joint of ankle and foot ensues, finally culminating into contracture. The true culprit producing the equinus deformity is the

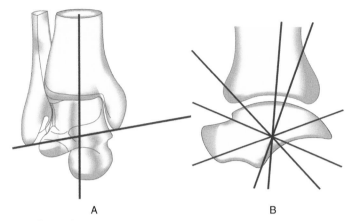

FIGURES 7.1A and B: A. Axis of rotation in coronal plane;
B. Axis of rotation in sagittal plane

tendoAchilles—spasm/tightness/contracture. If the equinus exceeds 45°, it is usually associated with cavus deformity of foot.

If the deformity is mild due to spasm or ensuing tightness of tendoAchilles, only physiotherapy, which includes repeated stretching of tendoAchilles can correct the early equinus deformity. If the deformity is severe, then surgical procedures like lengthening or subtotal tenotomy along with stabilization procedure or alternatively **Ilizarov technique** can correct the deformity.

MOTION OF THE FOOT

The equinus deformity is caused by shortening of tendoAchilles. Since tendon is attached to the calcaneus the deforming force is at the calcaneus. The rotation of the foot takes place at the axis of the ankle joint and; with the motion of forefoot, hindfoot also moves (Figures 7.2A and B).

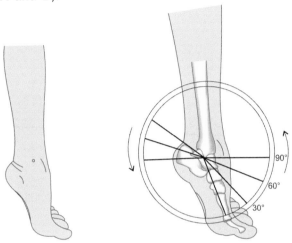

FIGURES 7.2A and B: A. Equinus foot; B. Motion of the foot in the circular direction

The lever arm from the axis of ankle joint to the calcaneus is shorter than the lever arm from the axis of the ankle joint to the forefoot, thus as per the mechanical principles, it is better to apply the force for correction at the forefoot rather than the hindfoot. Secondly, the force applied to the forefoot is the pulling force rather than the pushing force. As per mechanical principles, pulling force is preferred instead of pushing force. By adopting these principles, the equinus deformity is corrected by putting K-wires at the base of the metatarsals connected with the half ring and the pulling force is applied from the same forefoot ring. Further, for pushing the hind foot two K-wires are passed into the calcaneus connected with a half ring, which is joined with the tibial frame (Figures 7.3 and 7.4).

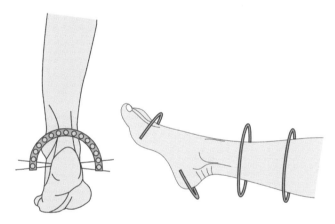

FIGURE 7.3: Half ring in calcaneus with K-wire

FIGURE 7.4: Location of forefoot, calcaneal ring and tibial rings

Relative Motions of Hindfoot and Forefoot

The foot (forefoot and hindfoot) moves in a circular pathway (Figures 7.5 and 7.6) with the axis at ankle joint whereas threaded rods move in linear motion. The circular movement of the foot is facilitated into linear motion by eight hinges thus the two relative motion have to be considered while correcting the deformity.

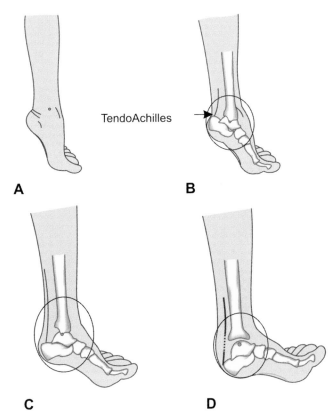

Figures 7.5A to D: By circular motion of the hindfoot for equinus correction. A. Equinus foot 60^0; B. Hindfoot rotation showing circle pathway. C. Hindfoot rotation $45°$; D.Deformity corrected

The movement of the hindfoot takes place while correcting the deformity of foot. Soft tissue contracture is responsible for hindfoot deformity. TendoAchilles lengthening by Ilizarov procedure is done by doing subtotal

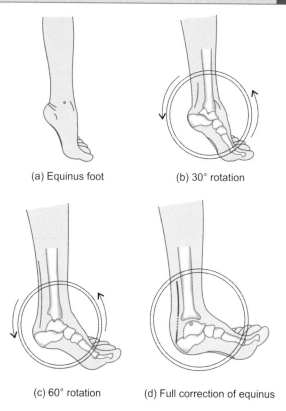

(a) Equinus foot   (b) 30° rotation

(c) 60° rotation   (d) Full correction of equinus

Figures 7.6A to D: Circular motion of forefoot with hindfoot. A. Equinus foot; B. 30° rotation; C. 60° rotation; D. Full correction of equinus

tenotomy of tendoAchilles either by two stab in which immediate lengthening is achieved and residual is achieved gradually or single stab in which incision is given one fingerbreadth above its insertion and then lengthening and regeneration are achieved at the rate of 1 to 3 mm/

day. As per the age of the child, the surgeon determines the rate of lengthening/regeneration. Younger children might require upto 3 mm per day whereas with increasing age it could be just 1 mm per day.

For achieving this lengthening, anterior and posterior threaded rods will have their excursion through their proximal hinges. The amount of excursion is determined by a mathematical calculation. For mastering this calculation, the relative motions of the hindfoot around its own circle and the forefoot around its own circle must be understood with clarity. Lengthening of tendoAchilles takes place around a circle, the radius of which is the distance from the center of the ankle to the point of insertion of tendoAchilles into the calcaneus OA (Figure 7.7).

Foot has a short leaver arm in the hindfoot and a long lever arm in the forefoot with fulcrum at the center of the ankle in the talus. When correction in the short lever arm of the hind foot takes place the resultant correction is reflected in the long lever arm of the forefoot by achieving the desired dorsiflexion. This dorsiflexion of the forefoot takes place around a circle, the radius of which is the distance between the center of the ankle to the insertion of the wire in metatarsal head OB (Figure 7.7). The measurement of the radius of hindfoot OB and forefoot OA is required for the mathematical calculation.

The soft tissue lengthening is represented by line AA' (Figure 7.7) while forefoot motion is represented by BB', e.g. if soft tissue lengthening is done @ 1 mm per day and the radius of OA is 60 mm and OB is 120 mm then

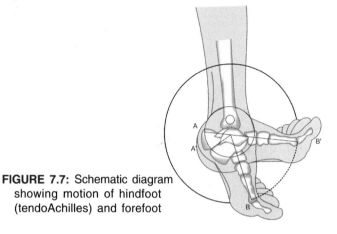

FIGURE 7.7: Schematic diagram showing motion of hindfoot (tendoAchilles) and forefoot

to get tendoAchilles lengthening of 1 mm the forefoot has to move 2 mm (Figure 7.7)

Mathematical Calculation for Deformity Correction

Basic Formula: Circle method for correction of 45° equinus

Arc length = 2 p R (a / 360)

OA—Soft tissue circle radius (r)

OB—Distracter circle radius (R)

AA'—Arc length of the soft tissue

BB'—Arc length of the distracter rod

a —Angular deformity

Arc length soft tissue = 2 pr (a/360)

r = 60 mm

And angular deformity 45°

Arc length AA' = 2 × (22/7) × 60 × (45 / 360)

= 47.14 mm

For the same angular deformity

Arc length formed at distracter rod is given by

Arc length (distracter rod) = 2 pR (a/360)

R = 120 mm

2 × (22/7) × 120 (45/360)

= 94.28 mm

Distracter rate (DR)—distraction is done per day at distracter rod when distraction at soft tissue is 1 mm.

D.R = (Arc length at distracter / Arc length of soft tissue) X 1 mm/day

= 94.28 / 47.14 × 1 mm/day

= 2 mm / day

Relative Movements of Anterior and Posterior Threaded Rods in Relation to TendoAchilles Regeneration

Movement of the forefoot takes place with the help of metatarsal rings whereas movements of the hindfoot takes place though the calcaneal ring and the metatarsal ring is connected with the tibial ring by two anterior threaded rods. Similarly the calcaneal ring is connected with the tibial ring by two posterior threaded rods. The rate of correction will depend upon the amount of tendoAchilles regeneration (see Figure 7.7).

Example—If the radius of the circle of the hindfoot (OA) is 60 mm and radius of the circle from the axis of the ankle joint to the distal hinges at posterior threaded rods (OC) is 90 mm and the distance from the axis of the ankle joint to distal hinges at anterior threaded rods is (OD) 120 mm then tightening of the anterior threaded

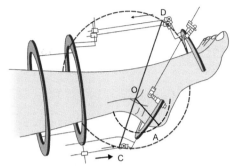

FIGURE 7.8: Schematic diagram showing relative movements of anterior threaded rod (OD), posterior threaded rod (OC) and tendoAchilles regeneration (OA)

rods will be 2 mm for 1 mm lengthening of tendoAchilles and the loosening of posterior threaded rods will be 1.5 mm (Figures 7.8 and 7.9).

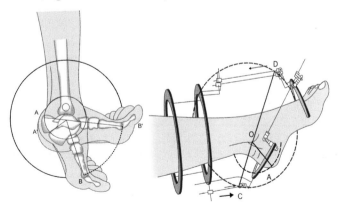

FIGURES 7.9A and B:
OA–Radius from the axis of ankle to insertion of tendoAchilles
OB–Radius from the axis of ankle to K-wire in metatarsals
OC–Radius from the axis of ankle to distal hinges in posterior thread rod
OD–Radius from the axis of ankle to distal hinges in anterior threaded rod

Table 7.1: Shows movement of threaded rods at various angle of rotation in comparison to tendoAchilles lengthening

OA	Lengthening of tendoAchilles in mm					
30	0.50	1.00	1.49	2.00	2.49	3.00
40	0.67	1.33	1.99	2.66	3.33	4.00
45	0.75	1.50	2.24	3.00	3.74	4.50
50	0.83	1.66	2.49	3.33	4.16	5.00
55	0.92	1.83	2.74	3.66	4.58	5.50
60	1.00	2.00	2.99	4.00	4.99	6.00
OC/OD	**Tightening of proximal anterior threaded rod in mm / loosening of distal posterior threaded rod in mm**					
65	1.08	2.16	3.24	4.33	5.41	6.50
70	1.17	2.33	3.49	4.66	5.83	7.00
75	1.25	2.50	3.74	5.00	6.24	7.50
80	1.33	2.66	3.99	5.33	6.66	8.00
85	1.42	2.83	4.24	5.66	7.08	8.50
90	1.50	3.00	4.49	6.00	7.49	9.00
95	1.58	3.16	4.74	6.33	7.91	9.50
100	1.67	3.33	4.99	6.66	8.33	10.00
105	1.75	3.50	5.24	7.00	8.74	10.50
110	1.83	3.66	5.49	7.33	9.16	11.00
115	1.92	3.83	5.74	7.66	9.58	11.50
120	2.00	4.00	5.99	8.00	9.99	12.00
125	2.08	4.16	6.24	8.33	10.41	12.50
130	2.17	4.33	6.49	8.66	10.83	13.00
Equinus angle in degree to be corrected 1°	2°	3°	4°	5°	6°

Examples: If OA is 60 mm, OC is 90 mm, OD is 120 mm and we want tendoAchilles lengthening (1 mm) per day; then tightening of anterior threaded rods will be 2 mm and loosening of posterior threaded rods will be 1.5 per day (at 7 am, 11 am, 3 pm. and 7 pm.)

FRAMES

Tibial Frame

Usually, it consists of two rings connected with each other.

Hindfoot Frame

Hindfoot frame consists of half calcaneus ring attached to the forefoot frame and tibial frame by means of threaded rods and hinges.

Forefoot Frame

The forefoot frame consists of one half ring connected with tibial frame by threaded rods and hinges.

Threaded Rods

Two threaded rods connect the forefoot frame to the tibial frame. These two threaded rods should be parallel to each other and horizontal to the ground. If the rods are not parallel, the motion of the foot may be hampered. Two posterior rods are connected between the hind foot frame and tibial frame (Figure 7.10A). Both these rods should be parallel to each other and horizontal to the ground. If the deformity is more than 45°, both anterior and posterior threaded rods will be proximally upward, the angle of both rods will be equal to cavus angle. e.g. if the cavus angle is 30° then upward angle of both threaded rods will be 30° (Figure 7.10B).

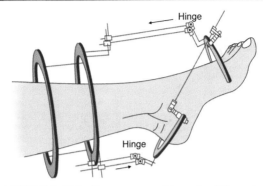

FIGURE 7.10A: Frame assembly upto 45° equinus

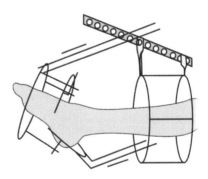

FIGURE 7.10B: Frame assembly for correction of equinus, anterior threaded rods connecting the forefoot and tibial ring placed in an angle in upward direction from distal to proximal, similarly posterior threaded rods placed in upward direction from distal to proximal

Hinges

Hinges are important component for deformity correction. In total eight hinges are applied for correction of equinus

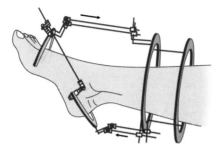

FIGURE 7.11: Complete frame assembly

deformity at various levels. According to the geometrical principles as soon as the motion of dorsiflexion starts the forefoot and hindfoot move in a circle with a base at the axis of ankle joint. This motion tries to bring the threaded rods in posterior or downward direction so loosening of hinges (constrained frame) is necessary for deformity corrections (Figure 7.11).

Constrained Frame

During correction of deformity, the posterior (downward) motion of anterior and posterior threaded rods are controlled by 8 loose hinges and after 10^0-15^0 of correction the position of anterior and posterior proximal tibial hinges should be adjusted according to the motion required. In case of tendoAchilles tenotomy the hinges should be loosened and tightened with every time correction, if they are kept loose it will interfere regeneration. In case of only soft tissue lengthening hinges are tight with nylon nuts, which promotes controlled motion.

Correction of Equinus (Figures 7.12 to 7.17)

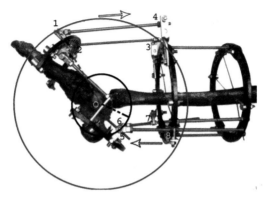

FIGURE 7.12: Foot equinus 45°. 'O' denotes axis of rotation of ankle joint, two anterior threaded rods and two posterior threaded rods, threaded rods connected with 8 hinges (1-8), all the distal hinges to be loosened and subsequently retightened after correction

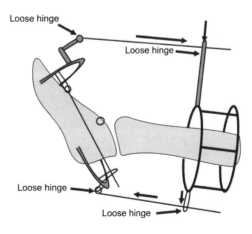

FIGURE 7.13: Constrained frame for 45° equinus deformity

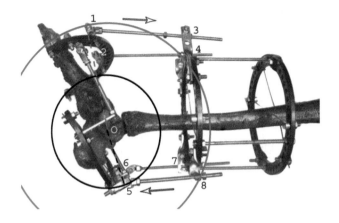

FIGURE 7.14: Stage 2—15° corrected
(residual equinus 30 degree)

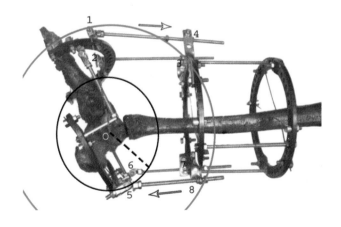

FIGURE 7.15: Stage 3—30° corrected
(residual equinus 15°)

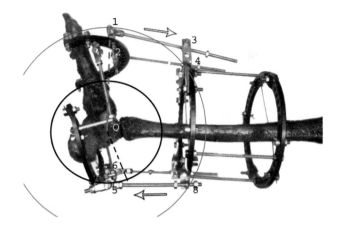

FIGURE 7.16: Stage 4—foot equinus completely corrected

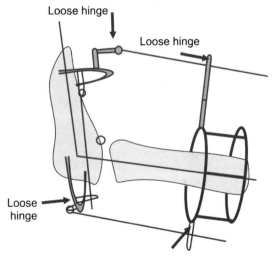

FIGURE 7.17: Constrained frame, equinus deformity corrected

Motion of Threaded Rods During Equinus Correction

During correction of equinus, it is important to know the movements of threaded rods. There are two motions in the frame, circular motion of foot rings and linear motion of threaded rods. The equinus is being corrected by tightening the anterior threaded rods and loosening the posterior threaded rods. The forefoot ring goes up whereas anterior threaded rods go posterior (downward), in the same manner, hindfoot ring goes forward and downward whereas posterior threaded rods go posterior (downward). The relative movement in between threaded rods and rings are controlled by loose hinges. After 10 to 15° of equinus correction the position of proximal tibial hinges should be adjusted accordingly.

Circular Motion of Foot and Linear Motion of Threaded Rods (Figures 7.18 to 7.21)

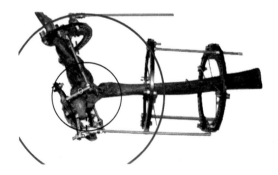

FIGURE 7.18A: Stage 1–foot equinus 45°. Bone model 'O' denotes the axis of rotation of ankle joint, anterior threaded rod and posterior threaded rod connected with hinges

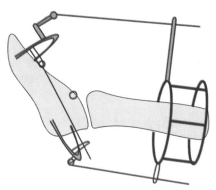

FIGURE 7.18B: Schematic view

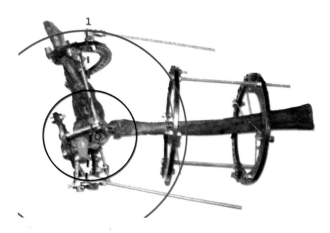

FIGURE 7.19: (Stage 2) 15° corrected (residual equinus 30 degree). Threaded rods going downward

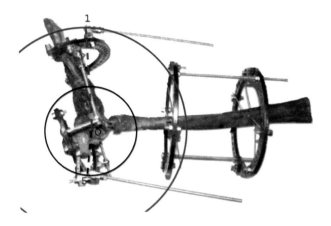

FIGURE 7.20: Stage 3—30° corrected (residual equinus 15°) threaded rods going downward

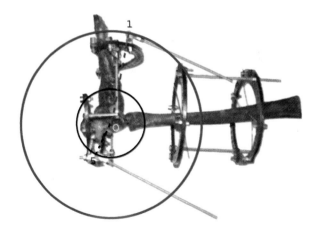

FIGURE 7.21A: Stage 4—foot equinus corrected threaded rods going downward

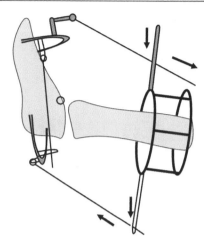

FIGURE 7.21B: Frame showing downward movement of threaded rods after full correction

Chapter 8

Precautions and Complications

ANTERIOR SUBLUXATION OF TALUS

Anterior subluxation of talus is a common problem that arises while correcting the equinus deformity at the ankle joint.

Normally the joint space of the ankle joint in lateral view is 3 mm, it has been observed that during correction of the equinus deformity this space diminishes. As soon as the space is reduced the dome of talus abuts on the anterior margin of tibia and the correcting force will displace the talus anteriorly (Figure 8.1). If the correcting force is further applied, it will distract the calcaneus causing distraction at the subtalar joint. If the space has diminished,

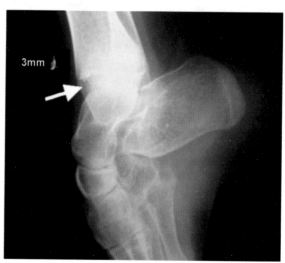

3mm

FIGURE 8.1: Preoperative radiograph of an equinus foot showing minimum joint space

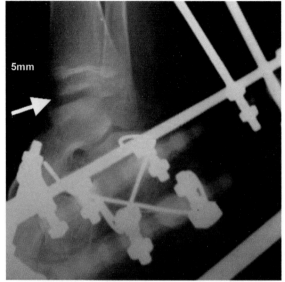

FIGURE 8.2: Postoperative radiograph showing distraction of talus before correction of equinus

then correction should be stopped immediately and distraction at the ankle joint should be done to achieve the joint space of 5 mm (Figure 8.2). The care of joint space and the shape of the heel should be taken simultaneously, because it has been observed that with anterior subluxation of talus, the heel also goes anteriorly during correction (Figures 8.3 to 8.5), X-ray of the ankle (lateral view) to be taken weekly.

It has been observed that if the equinus deformity is up to 45° then chances of subluxation of talus become less but if the deformity is more than 45°, then chances

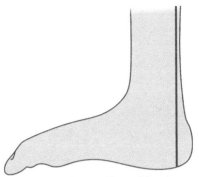

FIGURE 8.3: Normal heel

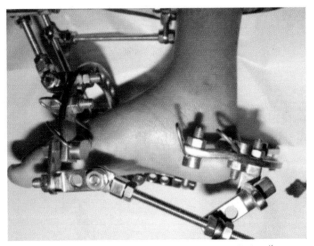

FIGURE 8.4: Shifting of heel anteriorly

of subluxation of talus will be more (Figure 8.6). The subluxation also depends upon the age of child, type of the deformity whether it is mild type of deformity or severe

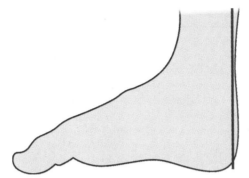

FIGURE 8.5: Sketch diagram (shifting of heel anteriorly)

type of deformity and it is corrected by distraction at ankle joint. In course of distraction sometimes the distraction takes place at subtalar joint instead of ankle joint then one K-wire is passed in the talus bone.

Method of Correction

Anterior Subluxation of Talus

There are two methods to correct the anterior subluxation of talus:

Distraction between tibial ring and calcaneus ring: Tibial and calcaneus rings are connected with three posterior threaded rods and hinges. The direction of the threaded rod is posterior so that motion of the talus will be posterior along with distraction. The distraction begins @ 1mm/ day till the anterior subluxation of talus is corrected and

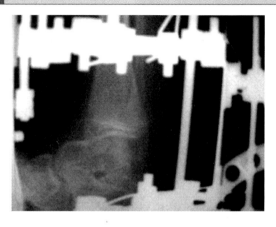

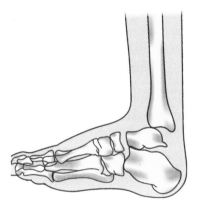

FIGURES 8.6A and B: Subluxation of talus
(*Courtesy Dr Anil Juyal, Dept. of Orthopaedic,
HIMS, Dehradoon)

a space of 5 mm is achieved between tibia and talus
(Figures 8.7A and B).

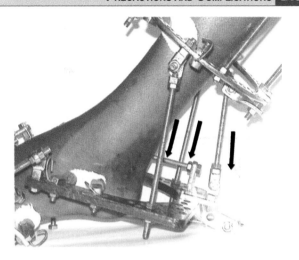

FIGURE 8.7A: Ankle joint being distracted
before correction of equinus

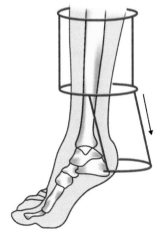

FIGURE 8.7B: Line diagram showing
joint distraction

Distraction between tibial ring and calcaneus ring as well as tibial ring and forefoot ring:

a. ***Configuration for distraction between tibial and forefoot rings:*** Tibial and forefoot rings are connected with four threaded rods. All the rods should be parallel to each other and the rods should be parallel to the ground. The disraction is done @ 1mm / day till 5 mm space is achieved between talus and tibia. It is followed by posterior shifting of talus by changing the configuration of the frame (Figures 8.8A to D).

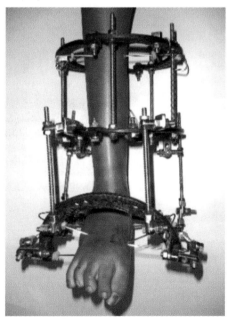

FIGURE 8.8A: Top view

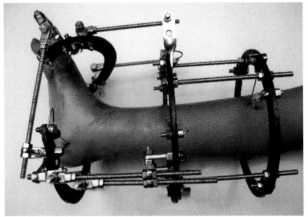

FIGURE 8.8B: Medial view

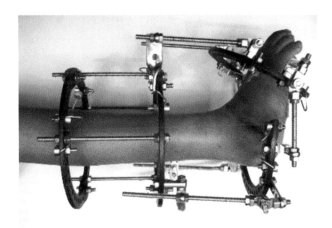

FIGURE 8.8C: Lateral view

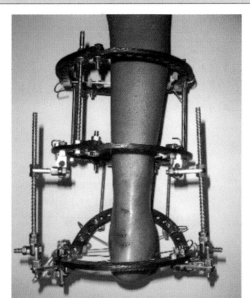

FIGURE 8.8D: Posterior view
FIGURES 8.8A to D: Frame assembly for distraction at ankle joint (distraction between tibial ring and calcaneal ring). All the threaded rods (two anterior and two posterior) must be parallel to each other

b. *Frame assembly for posterior shifting of talus:*
One 10 to 12 cm threaded rod is fixed to the anterolateral part of the tibial ring. The distal end of threaded rod is fixed with female post. The female post should be two-finger breadth proximal to the forefoot ring. One 8 to 10 cm threaded rod is fixed with female post, the direction of the threaded rod is vertical (anteroposterior). One hole male post is fixed

on the lateral part of the forefoot ring on the posterior aspect of the ring, second one hole male post is connected to the first male post, then a three hole male post is attached with second male post and vertical threaded rod, all the nuts are tightened.

A 10 to 12 cm threaded rod attached to postero-lateral part of distal tibial ring a female post is attached to the distal end of threaded rod. A 10 cm vertical (anteroposterior) rod is attached to the female post, the direction of the threaded rod is vertical (antero-posterior). A three hole male post is attached with lateral part of the calcaneal ring. One four hole male post is attached with first male post and vertical threaded rod, all the nuts are tightened (Figures 8.9 and 8.10).

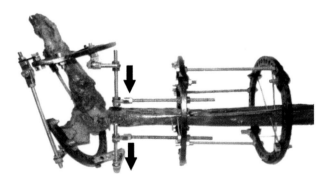

FIGURE 8.9A: Medial view

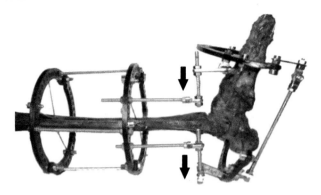

FIGURE 8.9B: Lateral view

FIGURES 8.9A and B: Placement of frame on a bone model

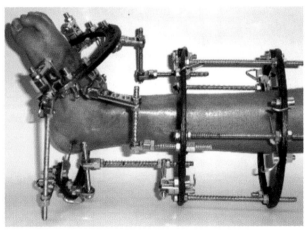

FIGURE 8.10A: Medial view

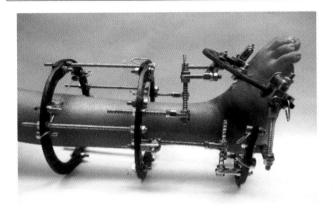

FIGURE 8.10B: Lateral view

FIGURES 8.10A and B: Distal distraction between two anterior and two posterior threaded rods. Frame assembly for posterior shifting of talus

The same configuration is applied in medial side of ankle joint.

Posterior shifting of the talus is achieved by distraction of all the four vertical rods @ 1 mm/day.

INCORRECT APPLICATION OF DISTAL TIBIAL RING

As a precautionary measure, there should be wide margin between the distal tibial ring and the forefoot ring. Distal ring should be fixed five fingerbreadth above the ankle joint (in an average adult) so that after correction the rings may not touch each other (Figures 8.11 and 8.12).

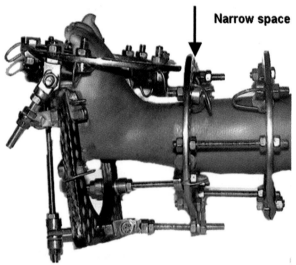

Narrow space

FIGURE 8.11: Showing incorrect application of the distal tibial ring

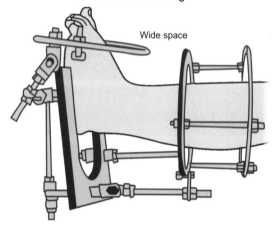

Wide space

FIGURE 8.12: Showing correct application of the distal tibial ring

FOOT RING NOT PERPENDICULAR TO THE FOOT

The foot ring should be perpendicular to the foot otherwise it will touch the shin of tibia during correction. Therefore either the correction should be stopped or the position of the ring be changed (Figure 8.13).

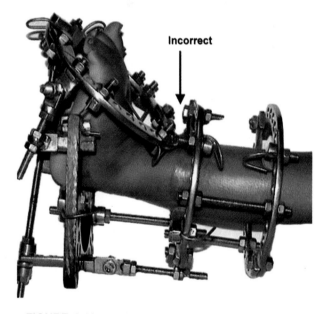

FIGURE 8.13: Ring is not perpendicular to the foot

STRETCHING OF SOFT TISSUE

During correction of equinus, there is stretching of soft tissues on plantar surface mainly flexors of toes and plantar facia. It leads to clawing of toes, to avoid this, toe support is given from day one (Figure 8.14).

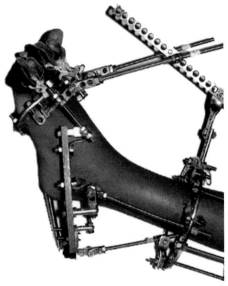

FIGURE 8.14: Showing toe support

Bibliography

1. ASAMI Group; Editors: A Bianchi Maiocchi, J. Aronson; Operative Principles of Ilizarov; 1991; Williams and Wilkins/ Italy.
2. BD Chaurasia's; Human Anatomy; CBS Publishers and Distributors.
3. Bagnoli, Paley; The Ilizarov Method; 1990; BC Decker Inc.; Ontario.
4. Calhoun Jh, Li F, Bauford WL, Lehman T, Ledbetter BR, Rigidity of half-pins for the Ilizarov external fixator Lowery R, Bull-Hosp-Jt-Dis 1992 Summer; 52 (1) 21-26.
5. Clark, Clark's positioning in Radiography; Ed. Tenth; 1979; William Heinemann Medical Books Ltd.; London.
6. Editor James B Stiehl; Inman's joints of the Ankle; edn. Second; 1991; William and Wilkins; USA.
7. Editor Peter L Williams, Gray's Anatomy; edn. Thirty-Seventh; 1992; Churchill Livingstone; London.
8. GA Ilizarov; Transosseous Osteosynthesis; 1992; Springer-Verlag.
9. Green SA, Harris NL, Wall DM, Ishkanian J, Marinow H. The Rancho mounting technique for Ilizarov method. A preliminary report/Rancho Los Amigos Medical Center, Downey, California/Clin-Orthop 1992;(280):104-16.
10. Green SA. The Ilizarov method: Rancho technique/Rancho Los Amigos Medical Center, Downey, California/Orthop-Clin North Am 1991;22(4):677-88.
11. J Tracy Watson, Steve Ripple, Susan J Hoshaw. Treatment of Complex Fracture; Orthopedic Clinics of North America 2002;33(1):99.
12. Muller ME, Allgower M, Schneider R, Willenegger H. Manual of Internal Fixation; edn. Third; Springer Verlag Berlin, Heidelberg 2004.

13. Paley Dror. Principles of Deformity Correction; Springer; USA 2002.
14. Pandey Sureshwar. Clinical Orthopedic Diagnosis; edm. First; Macmillan India limited 1995.
15. Vladimir Golyakhovsky, Victor H Frankel. Operative manual of Ilizarov Techniques; edn. I; Jaypee Brothers Medical Publisher (P) Ltd. 1993.

Index